Food, Power, and Agency

Food, Power, and Agency

Edited by

JÜRGEN MARTSCHUKAT AND BRYANT SIMON

BLOOMSBURY ACADEMIC
LONDON • NEW YORK • OXFORD • NEW DELHI • SYDNEY

BLOOMSBURY ACADEMIC
Bloomsbury Publishing Plc
50 Bedford Square, London, WC1B 3DP, UK
1385 Broadway, New York, NY 10018, USA

BLOOMSBURY, BLOOMSBURY ACADEMIC and the Diana logo
are trademarks of Bloomsbury Publishing Plc

First published in Great Britain 2017
Paperback edition first published 2018

Cover design: ClareTurner.co.uk
Cover image © ClareTurner.co.uk

A catalogue record for this book is available from the British Library.

ISBN: HB: 978-1-4742-9876-6
PB: 978-1-3500-8958-7
ePDF: 978-1-4742-9874-2
eBook: 978-1-4742-9875-9

A catalog record for this book is available from the Library of Congress.

Series: Cultures of Early Modern Europe

Typeset by Newgen Knowledge Works Pvt Ltd., Chennai, India.

To find out more about our authors and books visit
www.bloomsbury.com and sign up for our newsletters.

Contents

Figures

Acknowledgments

No project is written alone, in particular a coauthored collection of essays featuring a wonderful group of inspiring scholars and colleagues. This book would not have been possible without the generous support of the Fritz-Thyssen-Foundation for the Erfurt-based research group "The Eating Self," and the Alexander von Humboldt-Foundation for awarding Bryant Simon with a Humboldt Research Award.

The idea for this collection sprang from a terrific workshop hosted by Maren Möhring at the University of Leipzig. Thanks to Lisa Bogert, Anita Mannur, and the others, including the contributors, who participated in the event and contributed to our wide-ranging and ongoing conversations about food, power, and agency.

Thanks finally to Jennifer Schmidt and Clara Herberg and the rest of the crew at Bloomsbury. They have shepherded this project through every stage of the process from proposal to reviews to cover art to the final publication with great ease and clarity.

Introduction

Food, Power, and Agency

Jürgen Martschukat and Bryant Simon

In 1961, *Annales*, the leading and most innovative historical and interdisciplinary journal of the time, published a piece by the French philosopher Roland Barthes on the significance of food for understanding the past and the present. Trained as a philologist at the Sorbonne in Paris, Barthes argued that food served as a gateway, perhaps the widest available to scholars, to the grammar and semantics of a society. "Food *is* a system," Barthes declared, adding, "an entire 'world' (social environment) is present in and signified by food."[1]

Barthes pointed to three principle areas for potential food research, each a place where the operation of the larger system was revealed and could be studied. First, he stressed that food permitted a person on an everyday basis to identify him or herself as belonging to a nation. By consuming certain food items and by preparing, eating, and enjoying these particular foods in particular ways, people asserted who they were or wanted to be, and made known their political and national identification. Barthes suggested that in America, sugar was not just a foodstuff but also an "attitude," and that in France, wine was more than wine. He referred to foods like Coca Cola and *moutarde du Roy* as signifiers of national identity. While he might have relied too much on stereotypes and leaned too heavily on the nation-state as a unit of analysis, Barthes did see and identify the politics of food and the essential and performative acts of identification associated with food choices.

Second, Barthes talked in his *Annales* article about what he labeled the "anthropological situation." With this phrase, he pointed to the differences between people that were reflected by and shaped through food choices, consumption, and the making and growing of food. What people ate or how they ate it and who made it said a lot about how they saw themselves and how others saw them. It said a lot, in other words, about identity and perception, about race, class, and gender, and the everyday acts of making and framing these identities.

Third, Barthes pointed to the significance of food for health and the body and how it provided energy, alertness, and relaxation. This observation ties food to both the science of nutrition and the everyday in a myriad of ways. "Work, sports, effort, leisure, celebration," wrote Barthes, "every one of these situations is expressed through food." Quite obviously, food is more than a substance or a chain of chemical and biological reactions, though it is those things. "To eat," Barthes argued, "is a behavior that develops beyond its own ends."[2]

For a long time and with a few notable exceptions, Barthes's call at the dawn of the 1960s for a robust interdisciplinary, multiperspective food studies initiative remained unheeded by historians, sociologists, and cultural studies scholars.[3] Yet, in recent years, the study of food has become a booming research area. Scholars from a wide range of fields have explored a vast array of topics from the importance of food to colonization processes to the emergence of home economics, from studies of single commodities to investigations of national palates, from baby food to sushi, and from the McDonaldization of societies to the culinary triumph of apparent multiculturalism.[4] Yet the systemic investigation of how power operates in and through food has for too long been neglected.

This too, though, has begun to change. In her 2013 book, *Eating Right in America*, the food studies scholar and former chef Charlotte Biltekoff called attention to "how power operates through the seemingly mundane."[5] Two years later, in a study of food and identity, food and literary scholar Katharina Vester pointed to the need to understand the "Taste of Power." And in a 2015 article, historian Marcie Cohen Ferris, sounding a lot like Barthes, stressed that "food is history. Food is place. Food is power and disempowerment."[6]

If food, as Barthes contended, is indeed a system and embodies a social environment and a geography, a past and a present, and if food ties us to knowledge systems and the everyday and makes us explore differences between imagined national cultures and social groups, power then is a crucial ingredient in food and reflected by food. Exploring food as a system, really the manifold, complex, and overlapping relations between food and power, is one of the key goals of this book. It does so without applying a single approach, but through various methods, interdisciplinary research, detailed examples, and finely grained case studies. Digging deep into the complex workings of power embedded and layered in food chains, food production, food work, food choices, government food policies, food advice, tastes, flavors, and eating performances in different cultures and societies in the nineteenth and twentieth centuries, the studies showcased here make clear that conceiving of power solely as an instrument of coercion is too narrow. Neither is power an exclusive privilege of the state. Instead, power always entails multisided, and often uneven, relations between different human actors, institutions, beliefs, and things. The balance among these forces changes as situations change. Thus, power is dispersed and pervasive, overtly and covertly deployed, and embedded in and produced by the knowledge and truth systems of a society, that is, as Michel Foucault points out, in what is accepted as truth in a certain culture at a certain moment in history.[7]

Part of the power of food is that it is everywhere. It creates endless notions of good and bad: good and bad food, good and bad eating practices, and good and bad bodies. Good and bad food, eating practices, and bodies lead, as food and fat scholars Kathleen Lebesco and Peter Naccarato suggest with a nod to Pierre Bourdieu, to the accumulation or loss of "culinary capital." What we might call "food power" generates market value, social boundaries, and individual accolades. As Lebesco and Naccarato write, "Rather than assuming that culinary capital circulates in a fixed and predictable pattern, [it functions in . . .] multiple and potentially contradictory ways."[8] Therefore, food power is not only constraining and repressive but also enabling and productive, in the sense that it creates and structures possible fields of thought and action at every level and in every niche of society. It shapes relations, rituals, and reality, and individuals, identities, and bodies, and it challenges all of these categories and ways of thinking.

Thinking about the contingent nature of culinary capital and food power pushes the matter of agency to the surface. Widely discussed in the academic study of everyday life and in postcolonial studies, agency traditionally denotes a combination of self-reliance, self-will, and self-respect among historical actors who struggle against seemingly overpowering discourses, social relations, structures, and processes. Through their agency, historical actors use their cultural, political, economic, and social resources to make change. When it comes to food, meat packers have walked off the job, waiters have spit in soup, and consumers have boycotted unfair practices at their stores. In all of these seen and unseen protests, they deploy, with a nod to Barthes, an alternative grammar, different from the reigning order and way of seeing things. Agency then denotes the willingness and ability to confront seemingly overpowering discourses and structures, to rebel or write "hidden transcripts" of resistance, or sometimes to just walk away.[9]

Recently, this notion of agency has been amended. As a number of the articles in this book show, liberal societies expect historical actors to be in control of their own lives. These liberal societies rely on the principle that their citizens use their freedom judiciously and efficiently and present themselves as self-reliant and productive. Here, power does not work through constraining human conduct and outright coercion, but through incitement to be proactive. The prototype of a good liberal subject is someone who is busy, active, seeking to achieve things, in other words, someone who has agency. Therefore, agency is not necessarily and exclusively tied to resistance or withdrawal but also to compliance with the demands of power.[10]

At the same time, actor-network theory and the study of things, matter, and substances prompt us to continue to rethink the concept of agency and the power of actors. Again, food and the body prove useful here. As historian Chris Forth points out, fat, for instance, "has the capacity to assert itself, to resist or 'object' in its relationship with subjects.... As a substance, then, fat possesses the potential to thwart human intentions. Like any object, it can seemingly 'object' to our wishes as it pursues its own agendas."[11] In shaping his ideas, Forth refers, among others, to the work of the sociologist Bruno Latour, who himself has substantially contributed to the emergence of this wider notion of agency. Latour uses the term "actant" to denote nonhuman actors of various kinds: substances, things, artifacts, institutions that may exert agency as part of multiple associations and complex networks. According to Latour, human willpower is not the master of agency. It is of minor significance for understanding how these networks work, and, according to Latour, an actor should not be seen as the origin of an action but as someone or something that "is *made to* act by many others." Latour and actor-network theory conceive of the social as an endless number of flexible associations. In this assemblage, as Latour writes, "any thing that does modify a state of affairs by making a difference is an actor." Several essays in the present volume show quite clearly the role of nonhuman actors in the food chain. In one case, tragedy is triggered, in part, by pesky, difficult to control flies. Other essays show how running with or without an energy drink, or eating or not eating an ultragreasy burek makes a difference, even though the drink or the fatty food does not determine the action alone, just as the individual does not determine the action alone.[12]

Food, Power, and Agency explores the intersection among food, power, and different types of actors and forms of agency. It features eight essays by historians, sociologists, anthropologists, and cultural studies scholars from around the world writing about topics across the globe. But no matter the specific subject or exact location, each essay explicitly and deliberately explores and interrogates the power of food as well as the power relationships reflected and refracted through food. Each essay also carefully investigates the relationship between food and agency and how it embeds and hides power in specific political, economic, cultural, and social settings. The diversity of topics and locations explored in the chapters that follow makes the many modes of operation of power and agency easier to see. At the same time, they also make clear just how layered and textured these forces are in any given moment and in any given situation, especially when it comes to food.

The structure of the book and its parts are inspired by Roland Barthes's classic article cited above and the three major fields of research he outlined in it over half a century ago. At the same time, the book complicates and builds on Barthes's suggestions and agenda for food studies.

The book's first part, therefore, deals with food and the nation. The chapters by historian Leonard Schmieding on "German Restaurants in San Francisco" and by sociologists Rossella Ceccarini and Keiichi Sawaguchi on "Italian Cuisine in Japan" show how food is an agent of national identities and global cultural transfers and how it is employed by some to accumulate culinary capital. Schmieding describes how a diverse set of actors design urban restaurant spaces and utilize certain cooking techniques, dishes, and representations to speak to dining audiences. In this case, they transform ingredients and style into meals, a culinary culture, and a sense of "real Germanness." Ceccarini and Sawaguchi also look at "real-ness." They address the question of how Japanese chefs trained in Italy contributed to the spread of "authentic" Italian cuisine in Japan, and how power, agency, and prestige operated in a range of informal and formal nationally based and imagined culinary training systems.

The second part of the book looks at what Barthes called the "anthropological situation." Both essays explore how class, race, and gender interact in the world of food and eating and shape the positions and potential for agency of the players involved. In the first chapter of this part, cultural studies scholar Christoph Ribbat explores how waiters play central roles in contests for power and privilege in restaurants and literature. He presents the waiter as a highly gendered and racialized figure operating between servility and authority, which therefore helps us understand questions of power and agency in the culinary world and beyond. Ribbat also argues how, in this power field, waiters came out from the shadows by seizing another level of agency through writing their own stories. In these tales, the key actors are the waiters, who use storytelling to control and shape larger narratives of work and power. In the second chapter of this part, historian Bryant Simon takes us to post-Reagan America and presents a story of food, tragedy, and overt and covert state neglect in a chicken processing plant in Hamlet, North Carolina. Through this case study of one place, he explores the "capital moves" businesses make to assemble labor pools of tractable, vulnerable, and systematically silenced workers so characteristic of global neoliberalism. His essay shows the Barthes-like systemic links between economic and political power and how they transformed shop floor and community relations. Eventually Simon's story leads to a fire in 1991 at that Hamlet plant. Twenty-five people died there trapped behind locked doors. The managers of the factory and food health inspectors had decided together to close the doors. They were trying to keep out pesky flies, which threatened the safety of distant consumers and the owners' profits. The workers in the factory were again, tragically this time, made silent so that the voices of others would be made louder.

Following Barthes's suggested agenda for food studies, the book's third part turns to questions of food and health. Two of the essays in this part address the complex formation of healthy selves, while two others discuss transgressive acts of eating by looking at different types of fat, both as a socially made condition and as a substance. In the part's first chapter, historian Nina Mackert explores " 'Scientific Eating' " and one man's ongoing struggle to be a healthy and productive person. Focusing on Progressive Era America, Mackert shows how individuals tried to make sense of an increasingly powerful knowledge and dietary advice system where food choices and eating right were considered crucial to the creation of good citizens and a strong nation. Mackert focuses on a single actor and his diary to examine a painstaking and obsessive dietary regime. She shows how this person strained to transform himself into being who (and what) he thought he should want to be. This chapter, then, presents a human actor who is intertwined in a complex web of power fields and interactions, with knowledge systems, foodstuffs, and other nonhuman actors exerting agency by making a difference. A second chapter by historian Jürgen Martschukat on "Running and Eating Right in 1970s America" asks similar questions by addressing more recent fitness and health cultures. The essay explores how in 1970s America the pursuit of fitness was seen as a path to individual productivity, health, and happiness, and how exercise seemed to lead to self-mastery, success, and desirability in all walks of life. In this project, eating right, including the right things at the right time, was of extraordinary importance. Diet in general, and energy drinks in particular, promised to help runners become not only faster but also the "better" people they desired to be.

The third and fourth chapters of this part revolve around conceiving of fat. Sociologist Eva Barlösius researches the self-perception of bigger children in contemporary Germany and how being bigger is associated with deviance, moral failure, and an insufficient control over oneself. She shows how the body becomes a signifier of a lack of agency on the part of the individual, and how bigger teenagers develop an awareness of their externally ascribed deficiencies. In the part's fourth essay and the last chapter of the book, anthropologist Jernej Mlekuž explores disobedience in a story of teenage food consumption. In his article on eating ultragreasy bureks, Mlekuž discusses the most popular fast food in Slovenia and documents an everyday battle fought on street corners over the burek, pitting the young against the established order, and ideas of food as a source of pleasure against notions of food as morality. While advice guides and media figures have produced a powerful truth about the greasiness and unhealthiness of the burek, the burek remains, quite defiantly, an immensely popular food among secondary school students, looking for something to fill them up and as a means of resistance. For them, the greasier, the better. Eating an ultragreasy burek has, then, turned into an assertion of agency among Slovenian teenagers as they have taken power and endowed the transnational dish with new meanings and made consuming it a liberating and life-affirming act.

Together the essays in this collection take up Barthes's formidable challenge to put food at the center of historical, social, and cultural studies. They explore food as a complex and overlapping system, a system, though, that bends, breaks, and reconstitutes itself as actors—individuals, states, knowledge regimes, and nonhumans—exert their agency. That play—that ability—to create change or stop change through the combination of force, consent, and incitement is what agency and power are all about. And as this collection shows, these forces are always in operation when it comes to eating, food systems, and prevailing norms about health and healthiness and good and bad bodies. Food is not, then, so much unique as it is typical, typical of how power operates through the obvious and the mundane. That is what Barthes recognized and so will others, we hope, after reading this collection.

Notes

1 Roland Barthes, "Pour une psycho-sociologie de l'alimentation contemporaine," *Annales: Économies, Sociétés, Civilisations* 16, no. 5 (1961): 977–86. Cited here is the English version, "Toward a Psychosociology of Contemporary Food Consumption," in *Food and Culture: A Reader*, ed. Carole Counihan and Penny Van Esterik (1997; New York: Routledge, 2008), 30 (emphasis added) and 32.

2 Barthes, "Toward a Psychosociology of Contemporary Food Consumption," 33.

3 Anthropologists such as Claude Lévi-Strauss have also pointed to the significance of food as a gateway to the values, meanings, and structures of cultures and societies. Early historical works on food include Sidney Mintz, *Sweetness and Power: The Place of Sugar in Modern History* (New York: Viking, 1985); Warren J. Belasco, *Appetite for Change: How the Counterculture Took On the Food Industry, 1966–1988* (New York: Pantheon, 1990); Harvey Levenstein, *Paradox of Plenty: A Social History of Eating in Modern America* (New York: Oxford University Press, 1993). See also the sociological introduction to the study of food by Eva Barlösius, *Soziologie des Essens: Eine sozial- und kulturwissenschaftliche Einführung in die Ernährungsforschung. Soziologische Grundlagentexte* (Weinheim: Juventa, 1999).

4 To name just a few publications that have come out since 2000 and pushed the boundaries of food studies: George Ritzer, *The McDonaldization of Society*, 8th ed. (Thousand Oaks, CA: SAGE, 2014); Alan Warde, "Eating Globally: Cultural Flows and the Spread of Ethnic Restaurants," in *The Ends of Globalization: Bringing Society Back In*, ed. Don Kalb et al. (London: Rowman and Littlefield, 2000), 299–316; Lucy M. Long, ed., *Culinary Tourism* (Lexington: University of Kentucky Press, 2003); Gerard J. Fitzgerald and Gabriella M. Petrick, "In Good Taste: Rethinking American History with Our Palates," *Journal of American History* 95, no. 2 (2008): 392–404; Rebecca Earle, "If You Eat Their Food ...": Diets and Bodies in Early Colonial Spanish America," *American Historical Review* 115, no. 3 (2010): 688–713; Charlotte Biltekoff, *Eating Right in America: The Cultural Politics of Food and Health* (Durham, NC: Duke University Press, 2013); Helen Zoe Veit, *Modern Food, Moral Food: Self-Control, Science, and the Rise of Modern American Eating in the Early Twentieth Century* (Chapel Hill: University of North Carolina Press, 2013); Amy Bentley, *Inventing Baby Food: Taste, Health, and the Industrialization of the American Diet* (Berkeley: University of California Press, 2014); Katharina Vester, *A Taste of Power: Food and American Identities* (Berkeley: University of California Press, 2015); E. Melanie DuPuis, *Dangerous Digestion: The Politics of American Dietary Advice* (Berkeley: University of California Press, 2015).

5 Biltekoff, *Eating Right in America*, 8.

6 Marcie Cohen Ferris, "History, Place, and Power: Studying Southern Food," *Southern Cultures* 21 (Spring 2015): 3. See also Ferris, *The Edible South: The Power of Food and the Making of an American Region* (Chapel Hill: University of North Carolina Press, 2014). See also Vester, who writes that "Food is power." In *A Taste of Power*, 196.

7 Michel Foucault, *Power/Knowledge. Selected Interviews and Other Writings 1972–1977*, ed. Colin Gordon (New York: Pantheon, 1980). See also Michel Foucault, *History of Sexuality*, vol. 1, *An Introduction* (New York: Pantheon, 1978); Michel Foucault, "The Subject and Power," in *Michel Foucault: Beyond Structuralism and Hermeneutics*, ed. Hubert L. Dreyfus and Paul Rabinow, 2nd ed. (Chicago: University of Chicago Press, 1982), 208–28.

8 Peter Naccarato and Kathleen LeBesco, eds., *Culinary Capital* (New York: Bloomsbury, 2012), 2. See also Josée Johnston and Shyon Baumann, *Foodies: Democracy and Distinction in the Gourmet Foodscape* (New York: Routledge, 2010).

9 James Scott, *Weapons of the Weak: Everyday Forms of Peasant Resistance* (New Haven, CT: Yale University Press, 1985); James Scott, *Domination and the Arts of Resistance: Hidden Transcripts* (New Haven, CT: Yale University Press, 1990); Bill Ashcroft, Gareth Griffiths, and Helen Tiffin, *Post-Colonial Studies: The Key Concepts* (London: Routledge, 2000), 6–7; Alf Lüdtke, "Geschichte und Eigensinn," in *Alltagskultur, Subjektivität und Geschichte: Zur Theorie und Praxis von Alltagsgeschichte*, ed. Berliner Geschichtswerkstatt (Münster: Westfälisches Dampfboot Verlag, 1994), 139–53; Nina Mackert and Jürgen Martschukat, "Introduction: Fat Agency," *Body Politics* 3, no. 5 (2015): 5–11.

10 Nikolas Rose, *Powers of Freedom: Reframing Political Thought* (Cambridge: Cambridge University Press, 1999); Susanne Krasmann, "Regieren über Freiheit," *Kriminologisches Journal* 31 (1999): 107–21. For a forceful critique of some forms of agency studies, see Peter Coclanis, "Slavery, African-American Agency, and the World We Have Lost," *Georgia Historical Quarterly* 79 (Winter 1995): 873–84.

11 Christopher E. Forth, "On Fat and Fattening: Agency, Materiality and Animality in the History of Corpulence," *Body Politics* 3, no. 5 (2015): 51–74. Forth draws on Ian Hodder, *Entangled: An Archaeology of the Relationships between Humans and Things* (Oxford: Wiley-Blackwell, 2012).

12 Bruno Latour, *Reassembling the Social: An Introduction to Actor-Network-Theory* (Oxford: Oxford University Press, 2005), 46 and 71–2; italics in original.

PART ONE

National characters

No doubt the myth of French cooking abroad (or as expressed to foreigners) strengthens this "nostalgic" value of food considerably; but since the French themselves actively participate in this myth (especially when traveling), it is fair to say that through his food the Frenchman experiences a certain national continuity. By way of a thousand detours, food permits him to insert himself daily into his own past and to believe in a certain culinary "being" of France.

ROLAND BARTHES, 1961

1

The power of food: Immigrant German restaurants in San Francisco and the formation of ethnic identities*

Leonard Schmieding

Eating German in San Francisco

When Noah Brooks reviewed San Francisco's restaurant scene in 1868, he concluded that "there is nothing that is specially Californian. But it is a Californian specialty that here is daily set a repast, rich, varied, and inexpensive, and to form which contributions of nature and art have been brought from every land beneath the sun."[1] His judgment referred to the multicultural character of the City by the Bay. From its very beginning as a rapidly growing urban settlement in the wake of the Gold Rush, it had attracted newcomers from all over the globe. In his culinary experience, this peculiar diversity found its expression in a great variety of restaurants. Of the French restaurants, which set the standard of the time, he wrote that "French cookery is cosmopolitan as well as national,"[2] while the "Italian restaurants, however, are more exclusively patronized by the people of their own nationality than is true of any other class."[3] Chinese restaurants should "not be overlooked in any sketch of restaurant life in San Francisco," for the "Chinaman is liberal and bountiful to his guest; ... the skill and taste of the cook is exhausted to tickle his palate and gratify his eye, and a more changeful variety of courses prolongs the banquet than is ever found on the tables of any other people."[4] In terms of appeal, cookery, and customers, German restaurants seem to have ranged somewhere in the middle between the outreaching French, the exotic but hospitable Chinese, and the keeping-to-themselves Italian places. As Brooks described these places, "Germany has several restaurants—not especially distinctive, but essentially Germanesque in their customers."[5]

Almost a quarter century after Brooks's restaurant report, author Charles S. Greene's impressions from dining out in San Francisco's restaurants detailed what it was like to consume food in one of the city's German restaurants. "Here you may order prune soup or markklöse, may feast upon herring salad, Berliner klobs, a full variety of sausages, Wiener schnitzel, matzos (unleavened bread in disks a foot in diameter), and the waiter will not understand it if you don't want beer,—unless Rheinwein should be your fancy."[6] The food and drink on the menu were just as eclectic within this one nameless restaurant as the restaurant itself was within the culinary diversity of the city in its offering, at least in Greene's perception, a distinctly German fare to its customers. Palates in search of regionally and religiously marked meals, like the Wiener schnitzel or matzos, could become just as happy customers as non-German San Franciscans, who appreciated culinary difference and did not shy away from encountering other foodways.

The culinary encounter between the American consumer Greene and commercialized ethnic cookery of immigrants from Germany was not only characterized by eating and enjoying food marked and marketed as German but also, and maybe more importantly, by verbally communicating with the wait staff and using the written menu. The following episode of his experience shows how much his exchange with the waiter influenced the way he interpreted the food that he consumed. "At one place the waiter served me a pudding that I liked. I thought he called it *'Amorita.'* And though I wondered at the un-German name, I tried to feel duly sentimental while I ate the *'Sweetheart'* pudding. But one day I recognized it on the bill of fare: my sentiment had all been wasted, it was *'Arme Ritter'!"*.[7] Only after reading the menu and the description it gave of the dish could he clarify the misunderstanding—that he had eaten what is now known as French toast to consumers in America. He could obviously not follow the waiters' spoken German, for "in this restaurant you hear little English," but he just as obviously enjoyed feeling a little out of place: "The mildly pervasive odor of Limburger cheese salutes your nostril, and all you need is a view of a castle with a legend from the window ... to make you think yourself in the Fatherland."[8] The combination of the food served, the language spoken, and the atmosphere created allowed his imagination to transport him to Germany.

The examples of Brooks and Greene illustrate the power of food in crafting Germanness in nineteenth-century San Francisco. They demonstrate how power works as a productive force that people participate in when they prepare, market, and serve food, and when they consume, observe, and report about it.[9] It is in both the practice and the discourse of food that people—culinary actors in San Francisco restaurants—found the agency to negotiate the meaning of German food, and thus Germanness, in the City by the Bay.

My chapter examines the power of food in the formation of ethnic German identities in San Francisco at the turn of the twentieth century. In doing so, it investigates the restaurant as the site of this process. The restaurant lends itself to this scrutiny for two reasons: first, as food scholar Krishnendu Ray has shown, restaurants in the United States were mostly operated by immigrants and predominantly by Irish and Germans;[10] and second, the late nineteenth and the early twentieth century, witnessed the rise of the restaurant, when it replaced the tavern, saloon, and, to a lesser extent, the café as a semipublic gathering sphere of the ascending middle class.[11] Both San Franciscans and San Francisco Germans flocked to German restaurants in the city to take part in the construction of Germanness.

I analyze the German restaurant as an ethnic enterprise by way of two case studies, the Heidelberg Inn and the Bismarck Café. Zooming in on their engagement with food, atmosphere, and entertainment, as well as in their interactions with one another, I demonstrate how restaurateurs, waiters, and customers negotiated the meaning of Germanness and its significance for the city. I argue that it was these heterogeneous encounters that produced Germanness in the semipublic sphere of the restaurant.[12] Furthermore, I contend that although the Bismarck Café and the Heidelberg Inn offered a similar fare, two distinctly different versions of Germanness emerged in these two restaurants. While the Bismarck Café and its successors, the Hof Bräu and the States Restaurant, offered Germanness in a cosmopolitan context and were perceived as cosmopolitan in the San Francisco restaurant world, the Heidelberg Inn successfully achieved renown as an exclusively German place. In order to contextualize my food cultural analysis of Germans in San Francisco, I first describe the nexus between ethnicity, cuisine, and restaurants.

Ethnicity, cuisine, and restaurants among German immigrants in San Francisco

As the small settlement of Yerba Buena developed into the "instant city" of San Francisco in the wake of the Gold Rush of 1849, it attracted a number of immigrants from Germany. The newcomers from Prussia, Bavaria, Hanover, and other states of the German Confederation that were to become the German Empire in 1871 grew from roughly 5,500 in 1853 to over 35,500 in 1910. Together with their American-born children, their number totaled over 60,000, or 15–20 percent of the city's overall population during the early years after the turn of the century. They thus constituted a significant presence in San Francisco until they blended into the American mainstream in the wake of World War I, its accompanying anti-German sentiments, and Prohibition.[13]

Immigrants from Germany and San Franciscans of German stock, including German Jews, formed associations to maintain traditions they brought with them from their former home. They built churches and temples in which they could congregate and practice their religion among their coethnics, and they were active in founding businesses, small and big, that benefited from the city's open opportunity structures and contributed to its wealth as a Pacific metropolis during much of the late nineteenth and the early twentieth century. While associations like the *Schützenverein* (sharp shooters), the city's many *Turnvereine* (gymnasts), or the *Sängerbund* (choir) were rather exclusive in accepting non-German members, and churches, like synagogues, practiced a similar exclusivity in a religious manner, businesses in the urban public sphere served as the primary contact zones between San Francisco Germans and non-German San Franciscans. Especially restaurants functioned as transnational spaces of encounter, where Germans with different regional backgrounds and from different social strata interacted not only with each other but also, and more importantly, with other San Franciscans.[14] The majority of eateries operated by German immigrants as German restaurants were located downtown, employed mainly German staff, and offered both American food for lunch as well as German fare for dinner.

As German ethnic restaurants, the Heidelberg Inn and the Bismarck Café functioned as spaces of encounter. With their fare, their interior design, and their musical entertainment programs, they offered material culture and sensory experiences that were intended to frame the practice of dining there as distinctly German. What guests encountered, then, in the form of regional German specialties, served by German waiters, and in a German atmosphere, enhanced by German images and sounds, were fabrications of Germanness with which they were invited to engage. Regardless of their national origin or ethnic heritage, diners brought to this culinary encounter their own food practices, so that the meaning of Germanness that resulted from their interactions with and in the restaurant transcended any clear references to specific locales. Rather, Germanness, and specifically German food, came to exist in the third space between its alleged origin and its locus of consumption. The German fare as an ethnic cuisine was thus peculiar to San Francisco, as it did not exist in Germany itself as national cuisine at that time.

Even Germans who visited the Heidelberg Inn or the Bismarck Café therefore could not relate to a distinct German fare but only to regional specialties, and even those were heavily recontextualized and were only distantly related to everyday cookery in Germany in the nineteenth century.[15] But the ways in which the dishes were advertised, prepared, and consumed proved to be instrumental in crafting a sense of ethnic belonging in California.

Ethnicity as a social and cultural practice denotes the process in which historical subjects used power to create a sense of belonging to a specific group. As a process, it is ever changing and highly situational, and we as historians can only analyze its precarious manifestations, snapshots that allow us to zoom in on the phenomenon at a specific place and at a specific point in time. All we can gain from this snapshot is how historical subjects invented or even reinvented traditions in order to construct their cultural sense of belonging.[16] Who belonged to the group of Germans in San Francisco therefore depended on their changing social relations. In the context of their experience, they appropriated existing communities, cultural attributes, and historical memories by interpreting, adapting, and amplifying them. This process included enacting a change of relations from within as well as reacting to them, whether they came from inside or outside.[17] An example of this dynamic is how the German community in San Francisco changed in the course of World War I. Reacting to outside pressure, they ceased to express the specific markers of German ethnicity in the public sphere.

Cuisine as a social and cultural practice provides the rules and tools to work on ethnicity. More specifically, it equips actors with techniques and instructions to transform ingredients into meals and thereby achieve a culturally coded taste. Actors thus produce the self and the other, unite and divide people, and create culinary communities. The basis for this is not only what people actually cook and eat. The culinary other rather emerges out of cultural imaginaries, perceptions, and allegations of how other people eat. What follows for the analysis of ethnicity in the context of food culture is that the discursive aspect of cuisine as a social practice is just as important as its material aspect.[18] With regard to available sources required for any historical interpretation, this is all the more true, since cultural imaginaries are much better documented in written and visual form, whereas the actual meals are gone—quite naturally, since they were produced for being consumed in the first place.

The keyword for the advent and development of German restaurants in San Francisco around the turn of the century is cosmopolitanism. This term not only marks the emergence of ethnic cuisines as a result of mass migration to the Pacific metropolis and its open opportunity structures, for which the city prides itself to this very day.[19] It also stands for the rise of the middle class, who appropriated ethnic restaurants when it laid claim on public space during the turn of the century. Small-scale entrepreneurs, managers, bureaucrats, and urban professionals challenged the American moneyed aristocracy, who dominated the restaurant landscape with the French restaurants they frequented, which were inaccessible to the middle class, by celebrating what they termed cosmopolitan dining. At these non-French restaurants, they could consume a variety of ethnic dishes, free of aristocratic pretensions like French-language menus, multicourse dinners, and stuck-up manners. The emergent middle class showed that Italian, Chinese, and German food was just as good as French cuisine and thus laid the foundation for a more democratic restaurant experience in the late nineteenth and early twenty centuries.[20]

The meaning of cosmopolitanism changed just as much as restaurants themselves did in the City by the Bay during the first two decades of the twentieth century. Restaurateurs faced the challenge of rebuilding their businesses after the Great San Francisco Earthquake and Fire of 1906. They did so without much infrastructure to count on, and with competitors coming in from the south and the north Pacific coast. German business owners had to deal with another rupture when World War I broke out and anti-German sentiment gained enough momentum in 1917 to pressure Americans of German stock into hiding their German roots in public. For proprietors of German restaurants, who depended on selling German culture in the form of food and drink, this adverse atmosphere posed a big threat to their enterprise, and many went out of business. The ones who did not, changed their business strategy—sometimes subtly, sometimes radically. In the following comparison between two German restaurants, I flesh out how one restaurant, the Heidelberg Inn, was marketed and perceived as a German restaurant, which went out of business in 1917, and another restaurant, the Bismarck Café (1908–1911), respectively the Hof Bräu (1912–1917), was run as a cosmopolitan and German restaurant and merely changed its name to the States Restaurant in order to keep operating until the 1930s.

German "specials" at the Heidelberg Inn and the Bismarck Café

The Heidelberg Inn and the Bismarck Café bore a number of similarities: as new gastronomic establishments opened after the earthquake and fire of 1906 in prime locations both near the theater district around Market and Fourth Streets and the revitalized retail district, and as businesses founded and operated by German newcomers to the city offering a distinct German fare. The Heidelberg Inn opened some time in 1907 under the ownership of Henry (Heinrich) Louis (Ludwig) Hirsch. Hirsch, born in the Kingdom of

Hannover, Germany, in 1862, had immigrated to the United States in 1880. He first resided in San Jose, south of San Francisco Bay, where he operated a hotel and became a naturalized citizen in 1888, before moving to San Francisco.[21] The Bismarck Café was operated as a family business by Fritz Müller and his three sons from St. Louis, Fritz Jr., Charles, and Otto. They founded it after their success at the Lewis and Clark Centennial Exposition in Portland, Oregon, where they had run the German restaurant the Bismarck Café together with the local Weinhard Brewery, also a German immigrant business, from June 15 to October 1, 1905. In San Francisco, they continued their cooperation and served different varieties of Weinhard Beer exclusively at their new Bismarck Café.

In relocating to the City by the Bay, both immigrant entrepreneurs grasped an opportunity specific to San Francisco's situation after the earthquake. Many parts of the city had been devastated by the catastrophe, among them a great number of hotels, restaurants, and breweries along with their products. San Franciscans created a high demand for food and drink when they reconstructed the city, to which the Bismarck Café and the Heidelberg Inn catered. As newcomers without an established base of customers, Hirsch and the Müller family secured patronage of their businesses through active membership in the city's German associational life. Hirsch, for instance, served on the board of the Harmonie Singing Society[22] and helped organize the Californian-German version of the San Francisco Schwaben Verein's Canstatter Volksfest, the harvest festival, in 1912,[23] while Otto Müller, as a member of the Deutscher Verein, made the Bismarck Café available for a celebration in honor of Otto von Bismarck's birthday in 1911.[24] With networking activities like these, Hirsch and the Müllers gained valuable access to influential interest groups among German immigrants in the Bay Area.

When it came to offering and presenting food as German, however, their practices differed. Hirsch catered to customers in search for a German fare almost exclusively in German and thus made it difficult for non-German speakers, or people not familiar with German cuisine, to find their way through the menu. In contrast, Fritz Müller and Sons, although they sometimes featured almost the same dishes as Hirsch did, made an effort to be as welcoming as possible to a broader cross section of the city. In the landscape of San Francisco ethnic restaurants, the Heidelberg Inn therefore figured as a German restaurant, while the Bismarck Café acquired the qualifier cosmopolitan.

At the Heidelberg Inn, Hirsch and his employees featured both German and American dishes on the menu. The German ones came first, listed under "Heidelberg Specials" in German only. The only help a non-German speaker had was the distinction, in English, between the days of the week and between lunch and "Evenings." Consequently, these customers, if they were interested in German cuisine at all, had to reach out to the waiters, to other guests, or to connoisseur members in their party for the culinary guidance required to place their order of German specialties. The latter, contrary to what one would expect under the name Heidelberg, but in tune with the German theme of the restaurant, were not restricted to a southern German cuisine. Next to the clearly southern "Spanferkel, Apfelmus" (roasted suckling pig, apple sauce) and "Geröstete Eisbein, Kartoffelsalat" (roasted foot of pork, potato salad), one could indulge in "Hamburger Rauchfleisch, Erbsen Purée" (Hamburg-style smoked meat, pureed peas), "Kasseler Rippchen, Wein-Kohl" (Kassel ribs, cabbage/collards), or "Frische Blut- und Leberwurst, Sauerkraut" (fresh blood and liver sausage, sauerkraut) as well as the potentially Jewish but not kosher "Gefüllter Fisch, Rosinen-Sauce" (gefilte fish, raisin sauce) or "Sauerbraten, Kartoffelpfannkuchen" (marinated beef, potato pancakes/latkes). Hirsch furthermore encouraged his "appreciated guests to not hesitate in addressing the manager in order to make special requests for their favorite dishes."[25]

By thus reaching out to his guests, it was obvious that he preferred the interaction with German customers who partook in his specialties over American ones, although he did not exclude the latter. After all, Hirsch and his team also served American fare like beefsteak, sandwiches, and lobster. At the Heidelberg Inn, then, one could eat both kinds of food, but the manner in which Hirsch advertised them in his communication with the patrons suggests that guests with a German background were prone to consume fare marked as German, whereas non-German customers were more likely to order the American one, while they watched and observed Germans as the other.

A look at the menu at the Bismarck Café in the following illustration reveals how Fritz Müller and Sons advertised the restaurant's German fare in a much more accessible way. Among the "Bismarck Specialties," they made available dishes like "Hungarian Beef Goulash with Spätzle," "Hamburger Rauchfleisch, Deutsche Schnittbohnen" (smoked Hamburg meat, German green beans), or "Paprika Chicken with Rice," which appealed to northern German and Central European palates. But one could also find regionally marked specialties like "Wiener Backhuhn, Compote, with Lettuce Salad," "Kasseler Rippchen mit Sauerkraut," and "Westphalian Ham with Asparagus à la Vinaigrette" as well as the nationally marked "Deutscher Sauerbraten mit Potato Pancake" and "German Pancake with Apple Sauce or Lettuce."[26]

Only when the German names for the dishes were too hard to discern did Fritz Müller and Sons not bother translating them into English. Calling "Sauerbraten" sour pot roast, for instance, would have most likely deterred guests unfamiliar with German culinary idiosyncrasies rather than incentivized them to try out the new and other. The peculiar linguistic mixture on the menu provided diners with more guidance than the German-only menu of the

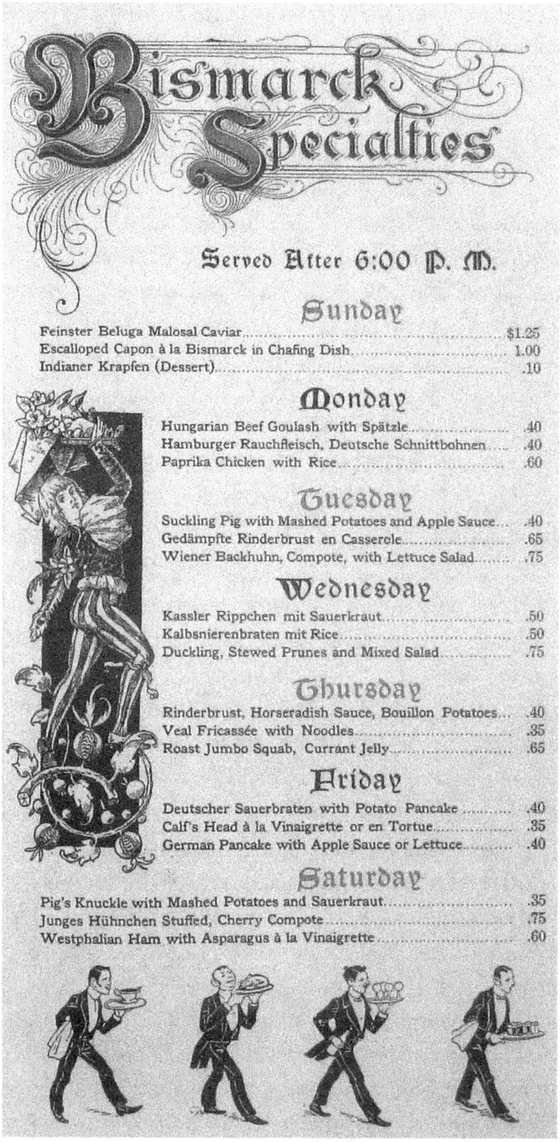

Bismarck Specialties

Served After 6:00 P. M.

Sunday

Feinster Beluga Malosal Caviar $1.25
Escalloped Capon à la Bismarck in Chafing Dish 1.00
Indianer Krapfen (Dessert) .... .10

Monday

Hungarian Beef Goulash with Spätzle .... .40
Hamburger Rauchfleisch, Deutsche Schnittbohnen .... .40
Paprika Chicken with Rice .... .60

Tuesday

Suckling Pig with Mashed Potatoes and Apple Sauce .... .40
Gedämpfte Rinderbrust en Casserole .... .65
Wiener Backhuhn, Compote, with Lettuce Salad .... .75

Wednesday

Kassler Rippchen mit Sauerkraut .... .50
Kalbsnierenbraten mit Rice .... .50
Duckling, Stewed Prunes and Mixed Salad .... .75

Thursday

Rinderbrust, Horseradish Sauce, Bouillon Potatoes .... .40
Veal Fricassée with Noodles .... .35
Roast Jumbo Squab, Currant Jelly .... .65

Friday

Deutscher Sauerbraten with Potato Pancake .... .40
Calf's Head à la Vinaigrette or en Tortue .... .35
German Pancake with Apple Sauce or Lettuce .... .40

Saturday

Pig's Knuckle with Mashed Potatoes and Sauerkraut .... .35
Junges Hühnchen Stuffed, Cherry Compote .... .75
Westphalian Ham with Asparagus à la Vinaigrette .... .60

FIGURE 1.1 *"Bismarck Specialties," Bismarck Café, Bill of Fare, © 1908, California Menu Collection, courtesy, California Historical Society.*

Heidelberg Inn. If curious newcomers to the kind of German cuisine that the Bismarck Café fashioned still needed assistance in making their choices, the menu signaled a general openness to further questions. It thus fostered the exchange over culinary culture between German waiters and non-German customers as well as between German and American guests, who interacted as neighbors at their respective tables in the restaurant and helped each other choose their meals.

At both the Heidelberg Inn and the Bismarck Café, the menu exerted power over the consumers in that it triggered microsocial interactions with other actors at the restaurant. It thus framed the experience of ordering food, which, in turn, involved appropriating the menu on behalf of the guests—a process of deciphering the bill of fare, interpreting the dishes, and imbuing them with individual meaning, as seen in Charles Greene's "Amorita" episode. Restaurant guests not only made sense of the written word and the graphic illustrations of menus. Dining out for them also included navigating the spatial configuration of the culinary location they chose to frequent.

Spatial dynamics

Just like bills of fare, restaurant spaces were first and foremost created by restaurateurs. Owners decided on a location within the urban setting, the interior design, and the visual decoration in order to produce an atmosphere conducive to preparing, serving, and consuming food. By appropriating the gastronomic entrepreneurs' offer, however, consumers contributed to making this space, not only by eating food but also by interacting with the location and the space of the restaurant. In the case of the Bismarck Café and the Heidelberg Inn, it was due to the consumer agency that the former became known as a more cosmopolitan place whereas the latter figured as the more German one of the two.

The Bismarck Café was located in the basement of the Pacific Building. Erected at the corner of Market and Fourth Streets, it stood in the center of the retail district and belonged to San Francisco's post-earthquake infrastructure reviving the downtown area. As the world's biggest concrete building, it housed law firms, doctors' offices, and other gastronomic institutions. The Bismarck Café could seat 1,500 guests when it opened its doors on May 2, 1908. The following newspaper report by Horatio Stoll, a San Francisco lawyer, published shortly after its opening gives an impression of the spatial organization of the restaurant: "The Market street entrance is down a broad marble stairway, through a wealth of tropical foliage where the men are relieved of hats and overcoats and the women given chance to arrange their toilettes. The main dining room, which seats about 600 people, looks like the heraldic hall of some German schloss."[27] Heads of dwarfs made of stone embellished the pillars of the vault, adding to the observer's almost fairy-tale rendering of the atmosphere (see figure 1.2). From his firsthand experience as a visitor to the Bismarck Café, it becomes clear how he interacted with the space that Müller and Sons had created. He reveled in awe of the German-made porcelain depicting the Iron Chancellor's head in profile, and he lauded the organization

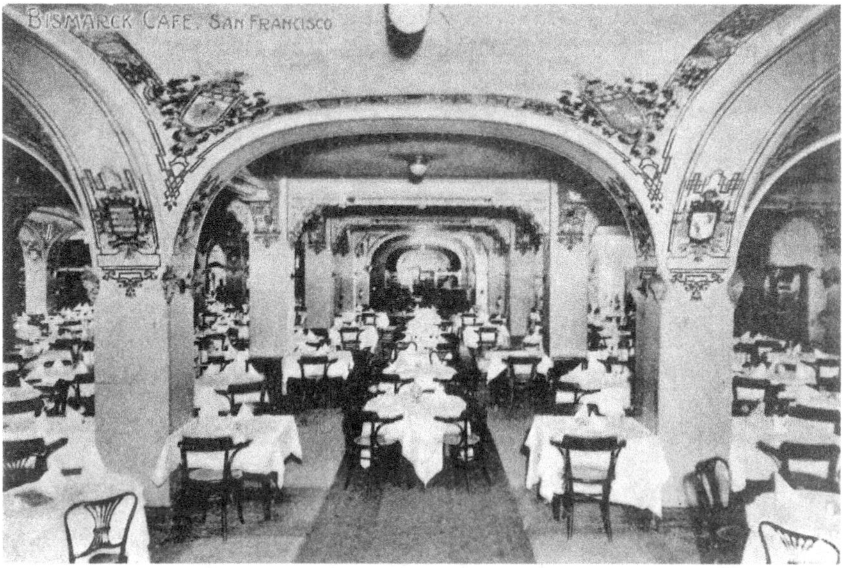

FIGURE 1.2 *Bismarck Café, Main Dining Hall, ca. 1908. Postcard in Author's Collection.*

of the space, especially the loges "where one can dine in semi-privacy and still listen to the music of the orchestra at the other end of the room."[28]

While Fritz Müller and Sons framed the consumption of German food with a German atmosphere in the main dining room, they had arranged other specially decorated places for the consumption of more American fare, including, for instance, the Beefsteak Room (see figure 1.3). "So called because here, in typical western cowboys' cabin, you can have a thick, juicy steak quickly broiled before an immense fireplace."[29] The massive restaurant offered three additional venues, each targeting a different clientele: the "Dutch cafe ..., a typical Holland garden on the outskirts of old Amsterdam," where downtown lawyers went for their lunch break; the "Louis XIV banquet room," which clubs and universities used for their banquets;[30] and the "university room, embellished with a series of bizarre French posters, grotesque caricatures of the arts, and some amusing hits at local celebrities."[31]

Catering to diverse tastes with highly differentiated spaces and practices of addressing and attracting their guests, Fritz Müller and Sons ran a successful business. They reached out to the nearby theater audiences with special dinner offer to draw in large late-night crowds: "The main cafe [was] comfortably filled about [by] 11 o'clock and a half hour later the scene was a brilliant one. The women were elaborately gowned and the majority of men were in evening clothes. It reminded one of the good old days before the fire when the Cafe Zinkand was at the height of its popularity."[32] Comparing the Bismarck to the

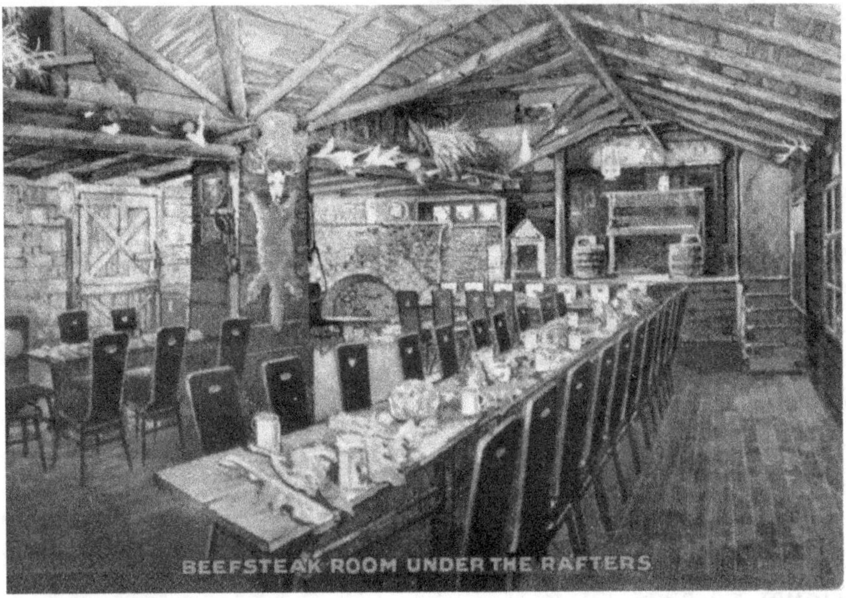

FIGURE 1.3 *Bismarck Café, Beefsteak Room, ca. 1908. Illustration. Postcard in Author's Collection.*

Zinkand was high praise, because it referred to the good life in San Francisco before the earthquake and fire. Others celebrated the German restaurant and its proprietors' contributions to reviving the downtown district: "The success of Otto Muller and his brothers Fritz and Charles in the management of the Bismarck since the fire has been phenomenal. While other cafe proprietors were hesitating about coming to the downtown district, the Muller brothers showed their faith by going in on a large scale and were amply rewarded."[33] They could even afford to open a new café, Muller's café,[34] and Otto Müller invested in the construction of the New Terminal Hotel in anticipation of the Panama Pacific International Exposition, which was to be held in San Francisco in 1915.[35]

All in all, the ways in which Fritz Müller and Sons integrated their business into the process of rebuilding the city and contributed to the revival of its restaurant and nightlife demonstrates how consumers perceived the Bismarck Café primarily as a cosmopolitan place in San Francisco. The diverse decor of the restaurant framed this cosmopolitan appropriation. Despite the fact that the main dining hall was clearly marked by both entrepreneurs and consumers as German, this was only one atmosphere among others, and it did not dominate the character of the restaurant.

Hirsch, in contrast, fashioned the Heidelberg Inn into a German restaurant. A look at the preface of his 1912 menu, in which he greeted his diners, shows how he organized his restaurant spatially and decorated it in a certain way in

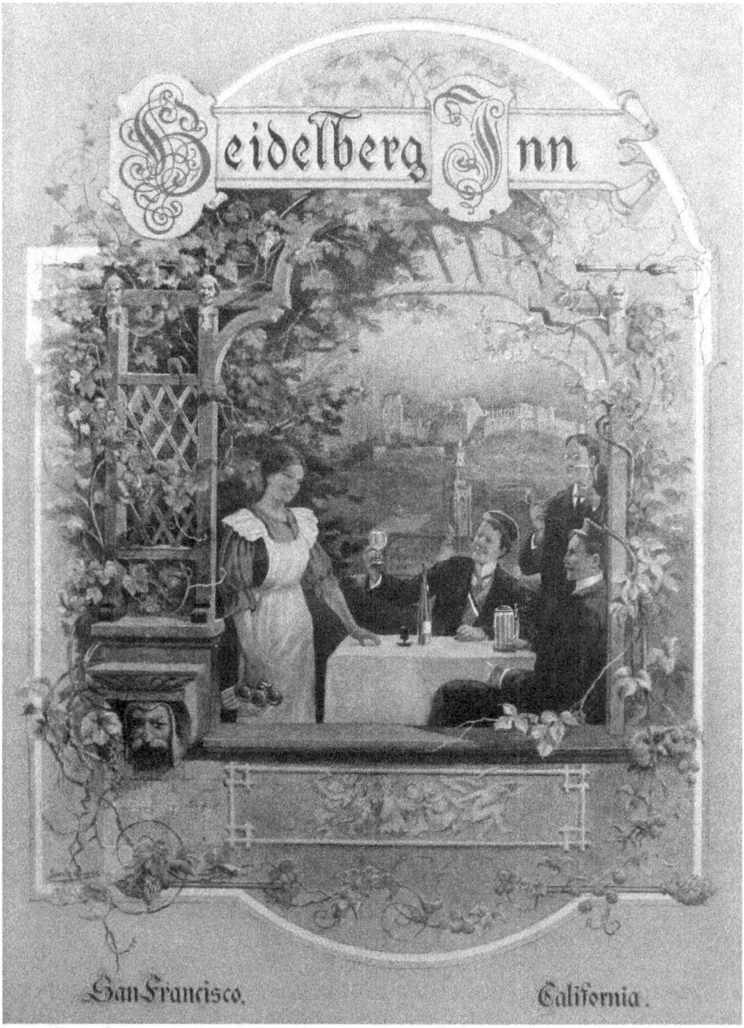

FIGURE 1.4 *"Beer Maid with Heidelberg Students," Heidelberg Inn, Bill of Fare, © 1912, California Menu Collection, courtesy, California Historical Society.*

order to achieve a German look and feel and how he used his power to prime and frame his customers' experiences. Just like Greene had done twenty years before, he invoked the term "Fatherland" to connote an imaginary trip to Germany that he promised to his visitors. The southwestern German city of Heidelberg, home to the oldest university in Germany, served as a place of romantic longing in his spatial marketing practice. Representations of the "Heidelberg student" and the "beer maid," both depicted in their "picturesque native costumes" (see figure 1.4 for a rendering of the bill of fare) greeted the customers at the entrance along with a glass mosaic of the "Old Heidelberg,"

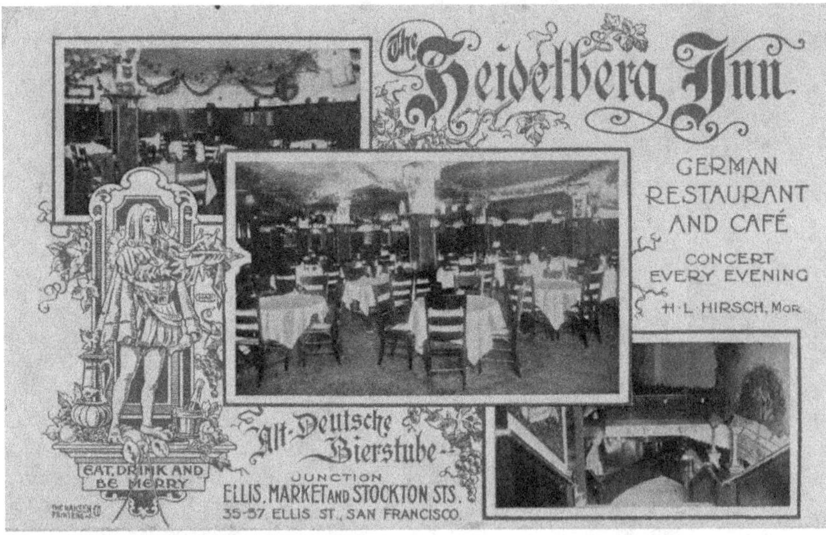

FIGURE 1.5 *Heidelberg Inn, Interior. Illustration. Postcard in Author's Collection.*

"this most beautiful of all castles" and set the tone for what kind of decoration was to be expected inside.[36]

After descending the stairs to the restaurant's interior, as shown in figure 1.5, customers would find several sections, all following the German theme: allusions to the different German regions, quotations from German literature, and images of German food culture. The booths in the "section reserved for ladies" were named after German cities and decorated "with a series of paintings portraying the history of wine culture." The main dining hall was dominated by a bar and booths bearing the "arms of the various German States" and "verses by the German poets." An "Old German Wine Room" marked by its "coziness" finished off this "distinctly German atmosphere."[37]

The Heidelberg Inn's combination of architecture, interior design, and visual decoration Inn conjured up, in the eyes of some of his patrons, the German atmosphere that Hirsch so praised in his menu. Among the few sources exposing how American consumers appropriated the space of the Heidelberg Inn, Clarence E. Edwords's *Bohemian San Francisco: Its Restaurants and Their Most Famous Recipes. The Elegant Art of Dining* documents the author's dining experience at the German restaurant in great detail. Published in 1914, it comprises the culinary experiences of someone who, as a bohemian by choice, wrote from the margins of society and simultaneously from its very center, being a lawyer by profession. Edwords could best be described as an early twentieth-century hipster with a peculiar interest in off-mainstream culture, which he chose to explore from his mainstream position. He represents the ambitious middle class, who challenged the monied aristocracy's claim on everything

European. His restaurant recommendation disseminated knowledge about ethnic cuisine in San Francisco and contributed to making foreign gastronomy more accessible for his social stratum. It illustrates how middle-class patrons, both German and non-German alike, appropriated the Heidelberg Inn, how they navigated its space, how they interacted with the offer of German culture, and how they thus negotiated the German theme of the restaurant.

In his bohemianism, Edwords liked the fact that one was left alone by other guests at the Heidelberg Inn: "Here everybody attends strictly to his or her own party."[38] It was here that he could enjoy "a camaraderie that has all the genuine, whole-souled companionship found only where German families are accustomed to congregate to seek relaxation from the toil and worry of the day." Servers who went by names like August and Heine attentively but not obtrusively waited on the guests, which consisted mainly of German families. "From Grossfader and Grossmutter, down to the newest grandchild, sitting and enjoying their beer and listening to such music as can be heard nowhere else in San Francisco, as they eat their sandwiches of limburger, or more dainty dishes according to their tastes." Like other restaurant observers before him had done at other German restaurants, he felt transplanted to Germany, just as Hirsch had intended, explicitly so in his address to his customers, and implicitly so with his decoration. Edwords continued his bohemian reverie: "One can almost imagine himself in one of the famous rathskellers of Old Heidelberg.... You have the real atmosphere, and this is enhanced by the mottoes in decoration and the flagons, steins and plaques that adorn the pillars as well as typical German environment."

It comes as no surprise, then, that the public perceived the Heidelberg Inn as a more German place than the Bismarck Café and other German restaurants of the time. Quite possibly, it did draw from a customer base of predominantly German stock, more so than its competitors, but it is impossible to determine this as a fact, since the register, which guests were requested to sign and "wherein are inscribed the names of many great and prominent persons," was not archived for historical inquiry.[39] Sources of popular ethnography such as Edwords's restaurant review, contemporaneous city guides, and newspaper reports help fill this gap. Since entertainment played such a prominent role in both operating and consuming the space of a German restaurant, the following focus on music, customs, and folklore reveals how consumers appropriated the Bismarck Café and the Heidelberg Inn.

Between the "Star-Spangled Banner" and "Die Wacht am Rhein": Music at German restaurants

The musical entertainment program also contributed to the German character of the Heidelberg Inn, as Hirsch made clear in his welcoming remarks on the menu. "A fine orchestra is maintained, playing the best of music, both classical and popular." People could dance, sing along, or interact with the orchestra in yet another way. According to Hirsch, they were invited to take part in a "hunting lodge custom," that is, to sound bells "in appreciation of the music," bells that hung over the "Stammtisch" and were attached to a "huge old knife" suspended from the ceiling. Another "feature of the 'Heidelberg Inn'," as Hirsch called this folkloristic practice, consisted of "a lion that will roar each time a new 'Fass' is tapped for the guests." Together with the spatial organization and the décor, the music program with its interactive elements framed the actual practice of consuming food marked as German at the Heidelberg Inn.

For the aforementioned Edwords, the icing on the cake of German culture at the Heidelberg Inn was the orchestra and its patriotic music: "It is when the martial strains of 'Die Wacht am Rhein' are heard from the orchestra ... that the true camaraderie of the place is appreciated, for then guests, waiters, barkeepers, and even the eagle-eyed, gray-haired manager, join in the swelling chorus." His observation not only proves that Hirsch, his staff, and his guests sang German music together but also that with this particular music, they took part in creating an imagined German community, militaristic and patriotic in nature. By performing songs like "Die Wacht am Rhein," Germans at the Heidelberg Inn excluded non-Germans, and at the same time, they contributed to the ongoing practice in Germany of utilizing music as a vehicle for conjuring up a *Großdeutschland*.[40]

To be sure, Müller and his sons also maintained an orchestra at the Bismarck Café. They even hired an Austro-Hungarian conductor to lead the orchestra, thus alluding to both German-speaking empires and the theme of a Great Germany. The music program—opera, operetta, and dance music—corresponded to the imperial theme of the name, the decor, and the atmosphere of the restaurant. However, this peculiar German kind of musical entertainment was limited to the main dining hall and does not seem to have dominated the overall character of the Bismarck Café.

The Bismarck Café displayed as much cosmopolitanism as it did Germanness, especially when it opened its doors for city-wide festivities, such as celebrating the New Year. On the occasion of New Year's Eve 1908, more than one thousand guests gathered at the restaurant. "Business and professional men, actors, miners, magnates, millionaires and successful men in all fields of endeavor," reported the San Francisco *Call*, "were the hosts, and parties of friends—as many as 25 in some cases—were seated together, with the wine the order of the evening."[41] The paper even printed the list of people who chose the Bismarck Café as their location to celebrate. It illustrated the audience's diversity: next to institutions like the German Consulate General and Union Iron Works, the prominent Jewish families Lilienthal, Sutro, and Levy were present as well as the renowned printer Louis Roesch (who had printed the Bismarck Café's menu) and the Anglo-American families Fitzgibbon, Murray, and Wilson. All of them were entertained by the orchestra's lead singer, who appeared clad in a "Stars-and-Stripes" dress when it was time for the countdown and started singing the "Star-Spangled Banner." They all joined the chorus and even overpowered the orchestra with their singing.[42]

Comparing "Die Wacht am Rhein" sung at the Heidelberg Inn with the "Star-Spangled Banner" of the Bismarck Café makes the contrast between them very clear: the former was not only marketed as a German place but it was also appropriated as such, whereas the latter served as a space for cosmopolitan gathering and celebration, with Imperial Germany being one of the themes of the restaurant. It should come as no surprise, then, that the Heidelberg Inn had to close in the wake of World War I, while the Bismarck Café could continue its operation, first as the Hof Bräu and then as the States Restaurant.

Transitioning into the mainstream: From the Hof Bräu Café to the States Restaurant

In spite of all their success, Fritz Müller and Sons had to close the Bismarck Café in 1911. They sold it so that they could concentrate on the upcoming Panama Pacific International Exposition in San Francisco in 1915, where they would operate, similar to Portland in 1905, a German-themed restaurant. Ironically, it was none other than Henry Louis Hirsch who bought the restaurant, had it refurbished to look like the Munich Hof Bräu Hofbräuhaus, and reopened it in the fall of 1912 together with his son Louis Henry Hirsch as the comanager.

Although the two Hirschs continued the German theme by supplanting the Prussian epitome of Imperial Germany with the royal Bavarian one, they also kept emphasizing the cosmopolitan character of the Hof Bräu. Instead of the German states on the booths customers could now find "private dining rooms bearing the names of the different states of the union," and the "university room" had been transformed into the "college room" (quite possibly due to Stanford University, Stanford and University of California, Berkeley using the room for banquets after college football games), "complete with all effects." Only the former beefsteak room was now called "Bauern-Stauble" (Bauern-Stüble), denoting a farmer's dining room.[43] The fare, although promoted as "real German cooking in true German style," expressed the hybrid character of the Hof Bräu. From the November 25, 1914, menu, patrons could order a number of German dishes, now listed exclusively in English, including

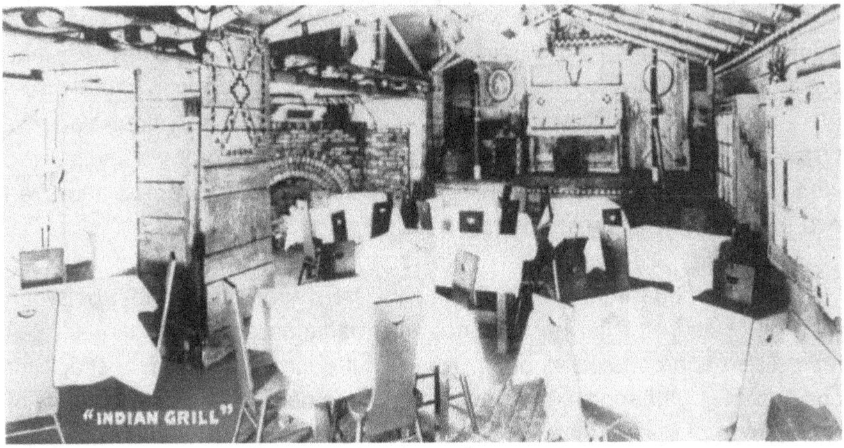

FIGURE 1.6 *States Restaurant, Indian Room, ca. 1918. Illustration. Postcard in Author's Collection.*

"German Cucumber Salad," "Pigs Knuckles and Sauerkraut," and "German Pot Roast."[44] The specialty of the house, though, was not a dish marked as German but rather Pacific abalone, a local specialty, which quite likely had been introduced by Chinese immigrants to San Francisco fare.

This cultural openness and fostering of cosmopolitanism proved to be an asset under wartime conditions and prejudices in 1917. While the Heidelberg Inn had to close, Hirsch junior, who had advanced to chief manager of the Hof Bräu, renamed it the States Restaurant, following a motto he already had established with the themed booths in 1912. When he could not run a business anymore by selling German culture, he sold American patriotism and marketed the restaurant accordingly. The Bauern-Stüble became the Indian Room, depicted in the following illustration, though the rest of the interior surprisingly remained unchanged, just like the bill of fare.

During the war, Hirsch advertised heavily in newspapers, bragging that he had invested in liberty bonds to support the American war against Germany, and that he had ordered his staff to speak English only at the States Restaurant, "the language of our country."[45] As a second-generation German immigrant, who had been born in California, he was in a position to operate the restaurant as an American entrepreneur, although it remained known to many still as the Hof Bräu.

Other than the careful and slight change in marketing the restaurant and the public display of American patriotism, Louis H. Hirsch did not have to adapt much in order to keep his gastronomic business running successfully. Whether this happened due to his agency as a versatile restaurateur or the less pronounced and less concerted anti-German actions on the West Coast has to remain unclear—it was probably a mixture of both factors.[46] Concerning the latter, Hirsch's interaction with the enforcement division of the California Food Administration in May 1918 demonstrates how this federal agency did not discriminate against him on the basis of his German heritage. After an inspector of the enforcement division had found out that the "Hofbrau (States Restaurant)" served bread without the guests explicitly ordering it, Hirsch was summoned to a hearing to determine the penalty for not complying with the food-rationing regulation. Neither his German background nor the fact that his restaurant was still listed as Hof Bräu played a role in this process. Much to the contrary, the hearing committee complimented him for running such a large restaurant so smoothly and appealed to his managerial skills when scolding him for his ignorance of the rules: "We have had Greeks and Italians up here who didn't know, but your case is entirely different. You are a man of brains." Greek and Italian restaurateurs stood in the focus of discrimination, whereas Hirsch managed to reduce his sentence from two weeks to two days by arguing his case with the representatives of the Food Administration.[47]

Hirsch and his States Restaurant survived the war as well as Prohibition and earned much praise in a retrospective on "Old San Francisco" in 1921: "We still have the States as a relic of the old Bohemia so representative of the golden age of San Francisco."[48] The accolade called it "one of the most universally and distinctive American restaurants on the continent," with its main characteristic being the "cosmopolitan character of The States' clientele."[49] And this cosmopolitanism, one might add, reached back to the Bismarck Café of the immediate post-earthquake period and resulted from open-ended interactions between restaurateurs, waiters, and consumers—interactions that invited, welcomed, and fostered a cultural exchange about the meaning of German food in San Francisco and its significance for the specific cosmopolitanism of the City by the Bay.

The power of food—the power of malleability

In my study of German restaurants as sites of ethnic identity formation in early twentieth-century San Francisco, I consider the power that people find in practices and discourses of eating and drinking to be instrumental in negotiations of the meaning of Germanness. I show how restaurateurs, their employees, and customers negotiated the ethnic marker of German in the practices of preparing, advertising, and consuming dishes listed as specialties at both the Bismarck Café and the Heidelberg Inn. While both restaurants offered almost the same fare, the Bismarck Café acquired a reputation as a more cosmopolitan place, whereas the Heidelberg Inn came to be known as the more German place. The prime reason for this contrast, I argue, is to be found in the different ways the proprietors fashioned their eateries. On the one hand, the Bismarck Café attracted a cosmopolitan clientele with its mixed-language menu, a diverse interior design, and a general openness with regard to music and entertainment. On the other hand, the Heidelberg Inn drew a more exclusively German crowd with its German bill of fare (for the specialties), an expressly German-themed interior design, and German musical entertainment, which fed into patriotism for the Kaiser and the Fatherland. Without their guests, however, who engaged with the food, the space, and the entertainment, neither of the two restaurants would have developed the way it did. Key to understanding how their Germanness came to be, then, is to analyze the consumers' agency in the processes of appropriating the restaurants.

The Heidelberg Inn and the Bismarck Café, as well as its successors, the Hof Bräu (1912–1917) and the States Restaurant (1917–1936), functioned as contact zones where historical actors negotiated the meaning of Germanness and its significance for the operation of restaurants marked and marketed as German. The restaurateurs exerted power to define Germanness by employing German chefs and waiters, by designing their menus to be used in certain ways, and by framing the dining experience with visual and auditory embellishments. The way the consumers utilized their agency to define Germanness differed, of course, from one individual patron to another and depended on their ethnic background, familiarity with German cuisine, and willingness to partake in the imaginary that these restaurants conjured. Unfortunately, the majority of voices that could document restaurant experiences in early twentieth-century San Francisco are lost to historical inquiry. What remains, at least for this chapter, are white American middle-class views, which, although well meaning and positive toward Germans (or at least their restaurants) in the city, fashion Germans as the other—at the Heidelberg Inn more so than at the Bismarck Café: Germans consumed different food, sometimes even undecipherable; they followed different traditions, as invented as they may have been; and they featured musical entertainment as an integral part of their dining-out experience.

The power of food in crafting ethnic identities—that is, the fact that San Franciscans and San Francisco Germans felt empowered to participate in culinary discourses and practices negotiating Germanness—primarily lies in its effect of presenting Germanness as extremely malleable. It was both Heidelbergian and Prussian, before it became Bavarian, and during all this time, it always included other German-speaking regions, so that it even conjured up a greater Germany. It functioned as a patriotic as well as a cosmopolitan space, and the States Restaurant, although it had retained much of its German fare, interior design, and music, was credited as one of the classic Old San

Franciscan American restaurants after World War I. The power of malleability inherent in practices and discourses of food, then, served to the advantage of the diverse German restaurant landscape in the City by the Bay.

Compared to other ethnic foodways in the United States, especially in the late nineteenth and early twentieth centuries, German food seems more powerful than, for instance, the food of Italian immigrants. While the latter greatly differed from American food, and Italian immigrants were encouraged to Americanize by changing their diets, German food was quite similar to an American fare, and therefore German immigrants did not have to confront such Progressive attempts at culinary and dietary assimilation.[50] Ethnic German food in the United States, or at least in the Bay Area, then, did not emerge from marginalized positions, but from a position of power.[51] Notwithstanding this privilege, it still had to react to practices of othering, as the different appropriations of the two restaurants have shown.

Notes

This work was supported by a fellowship within the Postdoc-Program of the German Academic Exchange Service (DAAD).

Roland Barthes, "Pour une psycho-sociologie de l'alimentation contemporaine," *Annales: Économies, Sociétés, Civilisations* 16, no. 5 (1961): 977–86. Cited here is the English version, "Toward a Psychosociology of Contemporary Food Consumption," in *Food and Culture: A Reader*, ed. Carole Counihan and Penny Van Esterik (1997; New York: Routledge, 2008), 32.

1 Noah Brooks, "Restaurant Life in San Francisco," *Overland Monthly* 1, no. 5 (November 1868): 473.

2 Ibid., 467.

3 Ibid., 472.

4 Ibid.

5 Ibid., 471.

6 Charles Greene, "The Restaurants of San Francisco," *Overland Monthly* 20, no. 120 (December 1892): 567.

7 Ibid., 568.

8 Ibid.

9 Katharina Vester, *A Taste of Power: Food and American Identities* (Oakland: University of California Press, 2015), 1–16.

10 Krishnendu Ray, *The Ethnic Restaurateur* (New York: Bloomsbury Press, 2016), 11–14.

11 Ibid., 64–6; Andrew P. Haley, *Turning the Tables: Restaurants and the Rise of the American Middle Class, 1880–1920* (Chapel Hill: University of North Carolina Press, 2011).

12 Maren Möhring, *Fremdes Essen: Die Geschichte der ausländischen Gastronomie in der Bundesrepublik Deutschland* (Munich: Oldenbourg Verlag, 2012), 17–21.

13 Heike Bungert, "Deutschamerikanische Ethnizitätsbildungsprozesse in San Antonio und San Francisco, 1848–1914," in *Die Deutsche Präsenz in den USA / The German Presence in the U.S.A.*, ed. Josef Raab and Jan Wirrer (Berlin: LIT, 2008), 59; Dino Cinel, *From Italy to San Francisco: The Immigrant Experience* (Stanford, CA: Stanford University Press, 1982), 17–19; Brian J. Godfrey, *Neighborhoods in Transition* (Berkeley: University of California Press, 1988), 58–61; William Issel and Robert W. Cherny, *San Francisco 1865–1932: Politics, Power, and Urban Development* (Berkeley: University of California Press, 1986), 72–9.

14 Jessica Ellen Sewell, *Women and the Everyday City: Public Space in San Francisco, 1890–1915* (Minneapolis: University of Minnesota Press, 2011); Barbara Berglund, *Making San Francisco American: Cultural Frontiers in the Urban West, 1846–1906* (Lawrence: University Press of Kansas, 2007).

15 Sidney Mintz, *Tasting Food, Tasting Freedom* (Boston: Beacon Press, 1996), 104; Konrad Köstlin, "Heimat geht durch den Magen. Oder: Das Maultaschensyndrom—Soul-Food in der Moderne," *Beiträge zur Volkskunde in Baden-Wuerttemberg* 4 (1991): 153; Uwe Spiekermann, "Europas Küchen: Eine Annäherung," *Internationaler Arbeitskreis für Kulturforschung des Essens: Mitteilungen* 5, January (2000): 31–47; Uwe Spiekermann, "Regionale Verzehrsunterschiede als Problem der Wirtschafts- und Sozialgeschichte. Räume und Strukturen im Deutschen Reich 1900–1940," in *Essen und kulturelle Identität: Europäische Perspektiven*, ed. Alois Wierlacher, Hans Jürgen Teuteberg, and Gerhard Neumann (Berlin: Akademie Verlag, 1996), 247–82; Hans-Jürgen Teuteberg, "Von der alten Schankwirtschaft zum feinen Restaurant: Streifzüge durch die Geschichte deutscher Gaststättenkultur," in *Gasthäuser*, ed. Herbert May, vol. 9, *Arbeit und Leben auf dem Lande* (Petersberg: Imhof, 2004), 27–54.

16 Werner Sollors, ed., *The Invention of Ethnicity* (New York: Oxford University Press, 1989).

17 Kathleen Neils Conzen et al., "The Invention of Ethnicity: A Perspective from the U.S.A.," *Journal of American Ethnic History* 12, no. 1 (October 1, 1992): 3–41; see also Russell A. Kazal, *Becoming Old Stock: The Paradox of German-American Identity* (Princeton, NJ: Princeton University Press, 2004), 1–13, and 272–81.

18 Eva Barlösius, *Soziologie des Essens: eine sozial- und kulturwissenschaftliche Einführung in die Ernährungsforschung*, 2nd ed. (Weinheim: Juventa-Verlag, 2011), 123.

19 Glenna Matthews, "Forging a Cosmopolitan Civic Culture: The Regional Identity of San Francisco and Northern California," in *Many Wests: Place, Culture, and Regional Identity*, ed. David M. Wrobel and Michael C. Steiner (Lawrence: University Press of Kansas, 1997), 211–34.

20 Haley, *Turning the Tables*, 1–18.

21 Henry Ludwig Hirsch, "Passport Application Henry Ludwig Hirsch," March 7, 1910, Passport Applications, January 2, 1906–March 31, 1925;

Collection Number: ARC Identifier 583830 / MLR Number A1 534; NARA Series: M1490, Roll 103, NARA.

22 "Aero Club Has Fun at Dinner: Members of Harmonie Singing Society Are Now Real Aviators," *San Francisco Chronicle*, March 10, 1909.

23 "Harvest Festival to Be Held by Germans," *San Francisco Call*, September 21, 1912.

24 F. Hagemann et al., "Zur Feier Des 98ten Geburtstages des Altreichs-Kanzlers Fürsten Otto von Bismarck," Invitation (San Francisco, 1911), BUS EPH, California Historical Society. The Bismarck Café thus anticipated the immigrant German and Austrian celebrations of their respective monarchs that the German House hosted after its opening in November 1912. The Deutsches Haus celebrated Emperor Wilhelm II's twenty-fifth anniversary in June 1913 and Emperor Francis Joseph I's birthday anniversary in August 1916. California Historical Society, SF EPH, German House in San Francisco.

25 Heidelberg Inn (San Francisco, Calif.), *Bill of Fare* (San Francisco, CA: The Inn, 1912). The German original reads, "Die hochwohllöblichen Gäste mögen sich nicht genieren dem Wirthe etwaige Wünsche für Leibgerichte kundzuthun" (translation by the author).

26 Bismarck Café and Catering Co., San Francisco, *Bill of Fare and Wine List* (San Francisco: L. Roesch Co, 1908).

27 Horatio F. Stoll, "Countless Comforts and Conveniences of the New Pacific Building," *San Francisco Call*, May 30, 1908.

28 Ibid.

29 Ibid.

30 "UC Berkeley Senior Men's Banquet," *San Francisco Call*, April 21, 1909; "Fifth Annual Banquet UC Berkeley College of Commerce," *San Francisco Call*, March 4, 1909; "UC Berkeley and Stanford Reunion Dinners," *San Francisco Call*, November 12, 1910.

31 Stoll, "Countless Comforts and Conveniences of the New Pacific Building."

32 Ibid.

33 "New Terminal Hotel Credit to Ferry District," *San Francisco Call*, December 31, 1910.

34 "Muller's Cafe," *San Francisco Call*, November 29, 1908, sec. 20.

35 "Insurance Building to Be in Classic Style," *San Francisco Call*, July 1, 1911.

36 Heidelberg Inn (San Francisco, CA), *Bill of Fare*.

37 Ibid.

38 Clarence E. Edwords, *Bohemian San Francisco: Its Restaurants and Their Most Famous Recipes. The Elegant Art of Dining* (San Francisco: Paul Elders and Company Publishers, 1914), 46–9. Unless otherwise noted, all following citations are from this source.

39 Heidelberg Inn (San Francisco, CA), *Bill of Fare*.

40 Celia Applegate and Pamela Potter, eds., *Music and German National Identity* (Chicago: University of Chicago Press, 2002), 1–35; Benedict

R. O'G. Anderson, *Imagined Communities: Reflections on the Origin and Spread of Nationalism* (London: Verso, 1983).

41 "Holiday Throng Jams Big Hotels and Cafes," *San Francisco Call*, January 1, 1909.

42 Ibid.

43 "The Picturesque Hofbrau," *San Francisco Call*, November 10, 1912.

44 Bill of Fare, Hof Bräu, November 25, 1914. California Historical Society, California Menu Collection.

45 Louis Henry Hirsch, "Some People Have Questioned the Loyalty of the States Restaurant Because It Had a German Name," *San Francisco Chronicle*, May 19, 1918.

46 Elliott Robert Barkan, *From All Points: America's Immigrant West, 1870s–1952* (Bloomington: Indiana University Press, 2007), 206.

47 NARA. The National Archives at San Francisco. RG 4, Records of the Food Administration. California Food Administration. Enforcement Division. Enforcement Records 1918, box 1, folder 1.

48 The States Restaurant Company filed for bankruptcy on April 9, 1934, and the case was closed on January 23, 1936. NARA, The National Archives at San Francisco. RG 21, Records of the District Courts of the United States. US District Court. Northern District of California. San Francisco. Bankruptcy Dockets, 1929–1970. 9 NS-S accession number 021-95-001, Box 7, Cause-No. 24572.

49 "The Who What and Why of Industrial San Francisco," *San Francisco Chronicle*, March 1, 1921.

50 Harvey Levenstein, *Revolution at the Table: The Transformation of the American Diet* (Berkley: University of California Press, 2003), 103–4.

51 Hasia Diner, *Hungering for America* (Cambridge: Harvard University Press, 2001).

2

Italian cuisine in Japan and the power of networking among cooks

Rossella Ceccarini and Keiichi Sawaguchi

Itameshi is a portmanteau coined by blending the words *Italia* and *meshi*, which in this context means food or meal. *Itameshi* refers to Italian cuisine that is either traditional or has been adapted to suit Japanese taste. Starting in the late 1980s, and intensifying during the 1990s, Japan experienced the *itameshi* boom. During this period, eating Italian food became trendy and fashionable, but at the same time, it was cheap and healthy. Until then, Italian cuisine had not been very popular in Japan.[1]

In the Meiji period (1868–1912), French cuisine represented the hegemonic culinary culture developed under the national policy of Westernization. For example, in 1871, Western diplomats residing in Japan celebrated the birthday of Emperor Meiji over a multicourse French dinner. At the time, the kitchens at high-end Western-style hotels in Japan, such as the Grand Hotel in Yokohama and the Tsukiji Hotel in Tokyo, were run by French chefs. By the end of the nineteenth century, less expensive eateries and restaurants would serve Anglo-American cuisine.[2] As a result, Italian cuisine was virtually unknown at the time.

To this day, many Japanese professional chefs continue to receive training in French cookery. The discovery of Italian food is often almost by chance. For instance, Tsutomu Ochiai, the most renowned Japanese chef of Italian cuisine, owner of the famous La Bettola da Ochiai in Tokyo, current president of the Association of Italian Chefs of Japan and an honorary knight appointed by the president of Italy in 2005, was trained in French cuisine.[3] However, after tasting Italian food, he decided to move to Italy, where he lived between 1978 and 1981 to master the local cuisine.

Typically, a boom has a peak and then fades away, leaving room for a new trend. Yet Italian cuisine in Japan has not been replaced by a new food fashion. It successfully battled the French hegemonic cuisine as a counterhegemonic cuisine.[4] Over the years it has become more and more popular in Japan as well as increasingly specialized, covering a wide range of regional Italian cuisines.

Nowadays, the Italian cuisine market in Japan is varied and caters to different wallets and tastes. There are restaurants promoting Italian homemade cuisine, stylish premises linked to fashion brands (e.g., the Armani and Bulgari restaurants), and family restaurant chains with dishes modified to meet local tastes. For example, the Saizeriya chain offers a standard fare, such as spaghetti alla bolognese but also offers a local version of pasta garnished with seaweed and spicy *tarako* sauce (cod roe sauce).

Moreover, Japanese-Italian restaurants are expanding overseas. In recent years, Saizeriya opened outlets in China and Singapore and a plant in Australia to manufacture frozen and chilled Italian food. The first Capricciosa restaurant was opened in Tokyo in 1978 by head chef Masaaki Honda, who had received his training in Italy in 1962. Now the company has 140 outlets all over the Japanese archipelago as well as restaurants in Guam, Malaysia, the Philippines, and Singapore.

Meanwhile, Salvatore Cuomo, an Italian-born chef, brought Napoli-style pizza from Italy to Japan and then reexported it across Asia. In the 1980s, Cuomo moved to Japan with his family. By 1995, thanks to the runaway success of Ristorante da Salvatore, he was scouted by the Y's Table Corporation to set up and manage, among various establishments, Salvatore Cuomo Brothers and Pizza Salvatore Cuomo. Currently, he has restaurants across Japan and in Seoul, Shanghai, and Taipei, and is involved in training Chinese and Korean *pizzaiolos* (pizza makers). He regularly takes the most talented of his students to Naples. In 2008, he was featured in the Italian news when participating in the Napoli Pizza Fest Competition with his team of twenty-five Japanese and six Chinese contestants.

Surely, there are many factors that have contributed to the success of Italian restaurants in Japan. A few of the most significant contributing factors are a general interest in products "Made in Italy," the liberalization of overseas travel in 1964, and the expanding number of consumers with more time and money to travel and experience new food as well as the end of the bubble economy era that made French cuisine seem too expensive. Also, we cannot underestimate the role played by the Japanese born in the 1960s, who supported Italian cuisine as a countercuisine to the hegemonic French.

Still, it would have been impossible to respond to the growing demand for Italian cuisine without the existence of a number of Italian-trained chefs in Japan or without a training system built over the years to create a network of culinary professionals.

The aim of this chapter is to shed light on the process that established Italian cuisine in Japan, first, as countercuisine and then, as a widely popular and favorite fare on the country's culinary scene. Particularly, the focus is on Japanese individuals who moved to Italy to receive gastronomic training, thus acquiring valuable job skills and establishing a network of culinary and social knowledge not only in Japan but also between the two countries. In doing so, the chapter utilizes a positive and productive notion of power.

As noted by Derek Gregory et al., the concept of power, broadly defined is the ability of one agent to affect the actions or attitudes of another. Usually, it has a negative connotation. However, they argue,

> It is trite to think of power only in negative terms. The possibility of having a conversation with someone, of running a class or seminar in which people can learn, of playing a football match, depends upon the deployment of power: of people taking turns to speak and listen, of students and teachers doing work as agreed, of players deferring to a referee. People both exercise power and are on the receiving end of power at different times every day, in all realms of life. More important than the fact that power is exercised is the way in which power is constructed and deployed.[5]

This chapter addresses the power held by Japanese chefs trained in Italy in making popular Italian cuisine in Japan, a power that has been constructed and deployed through the aid of a variety of informal and semiformal training systems. Together, these provided cooks with kitchen and cooking skills but also with powerful cultural and social capital that moved them from a status of power receivers to a status of power holders.[6]

This chapter starts with an overview of the multifaceted Italian cuisine as it has been constructed both in Italy and abroad. Then it presents a short history of Italian cuisine in Japan, highlighting the *shugyo* (training system) of chefs and of artisanal pizza makers.

Italian cuisine at home and away

Italy is often described as the land of a thousand bell towers. The campanile (bell tower) is a traditional landmark in every town. It is a symbol of belonging. Italian students of anthropology are often familiar with the account of the Campanile of Marcellinara, a small township in the southern Calabria region.

The scholar Ernesto De Martino was visiting the area with his associates in the 1960s. The group had been driving through the area, but they were unfamiliar with the roads. They were relieved when they ran across an old shepherd at a crossroad. Finding it difficult to understand the information given by the old man, they asked him to join them and show them the way, promising to drive him back. The shepherd agreed, albeit reluctantly. However, his expression became terrified as soon as he lost sight of the campanile. He looked so frightened that the group decided to take him back to the starting point immediately. The shepherd continued to look out the window, and his face gained serenity only when the campanile appeared again. The man felt lost when he lost sight of the bell tower, which represented his whole world.[7]

The Italian expression *campanilismo* originates from the word campanile. As pointed out by Fabio Parasecoli,

> This profoundly Italian expression refers to the love, pride and attachment to a certain place by those whose homes are located in the area metaphorically covered by the shadow of the bell tower. *Campanilismo* expresses itself through food as well. Towns, cities and even tiny countryside or mountain villages boast traditions that are unique or shared only with the immediate surrounding territory, often reflecting artisanal skills and rural civilizations that are visibly changing and, some say, slowly disappearing.[8]

This diversity is evident even in Italian food vocabulary. Thousands of lemmas fall under the category of pasta. Philologist Franco Mosino has recorded 1,238 names designating pasta.[9] In 1909, Vittorio Agnetti, a medical practitioner, drafted a unique book containing recipes classified according to the different regions. In his short preface, Agnetti wrote,

> Italy, due to the centuries-old divisions endured by the regions, has diverse and varied customs and traditions; among which eating habits cannot be disregarded. That is why, from the inhabitants of Friuli (claiming German ancestry) to the inhabitants of Sicily (claiming Arabian ancestry), there is among us a multiplicity of body types as well as culinary lifestyles. The recipes of the dishes that we have been able to collect, with considerable amount of patience, reflect this diversity. Moreover, gathered together, we may say that they disclose unknown treasures, unheard of by the majority of us. They demonstrate how our national cuisine, albeit almost unknown, due to its variety and delectability, overcomes the very well-known French cuisine by far.[10]

Given this diversity, acknowledged more than one hundred years ago yet almost forgotten during the era of Italian industrialization, should we be talking about Italian cuisine today? Indeed, there are common traits even in the diverse food and culinary habits scattered all over the peninsula. For instance, the idea of a healthy and simple cuisine consisting of a few ingredients expertly combined to emphasize essential flavors is common to the different styles of the North and the South. Over the last hundred years, a variety of books focusing on the different dishes and culinary methods have promoted the idea of a cuisine belonging to Italy as a whole. Among these works, the most popular is *La scienza in cucina e l'arte di mangiar bene* (*Science in the Kitchen and the Art of Eating Well*). First published in 1891, this recipe book written by Pellegrino Artusi addressed average middle-class readers rather than professional cooks, and it became the unifying symbol of Italian gastronomy. As noted by food historian Massimo Montanari, the local diversity itself represented one of the primary features of Italian cuisine.[11]

While tasting today's Italian cuisine in all its variety around the world, we enjoy the fruits of the Italian unification processes, military diet, fascism, technological changes, and other sociohistorical events, among which migration has played crucial and multiple roles. Italian migrants brought their food outside of Italian boundaries, and, once beyond these boundaries, they helped construct the idea of a unified Italian cuisine.[12] They even contributed to the development of new local foods, such as the New Orleans muffuletta sandwich, the name and origin of which bear witness to the Sicilian migrants who worked on the sugar-cane and cotton plantations of Louisiana during the nineteenth century.[13] The role of Italian migrants and their pattern of opening food frontiers that originally catered to their own community and then to the locals have been widely studied. Scholars have paid attention to the spread of Italian cuisine and to the role played by the Italian communities in America,[14] in Australia,[15] and in Europe.[16] It is as though through different paths, Italian cuisine has been able to climb the culinary ladder from being the food of the poor migrant to becoming a cuisine imbued with high social status, a cuisine to be enjoyed in humble premises as well as in expensive restaurants.

Ulrike Thoms points out that, at least in Germany, the critical feature for the popularization of Italian cuisine "was not the actual movements of migration and the raw number of immigrants but the strength of the ethnic economies and networks they built."[17] This is something that we have to bear in mind when looking at the path of Italian cuisine in Japan. The Italian community in Japan has always been smaller in comparison to that in the Americas and Europe. In the 1990s, at the peak of the *itameshi* boom, there were only 900 Italians registered in Japan under the Alien Registration Law, compared, for instance, to 3,606 Germans; 3,166 French; and 10,206 Britons.[18] Indeed, in order to analyze the development of Italian cuisine in Japan, we have to look at networks. However, this does not refer to a general network of migrants but rather to a specific set of connections between Italian and Japanese chefs and restaurant workers.

Italian cuisine and Japan

You do not have to be a keen observer to notice that food plays a prominent role in the Japanese culture. Bookshop shelves are filled with cookbooks and culinary tales, and food is omnipresent on Japanese television. In fact, Japan gave birth to *Ryori no Tetsujin*, the popular culinary show globally known as *The Iron Chef*. Food is ubiquitous on Japanese television, and is represented on just about every program. For example, a travel show will not miss a stopover at the best restaurant in town; a general entertainment show will have guests talking about food or indulging in a gourmet experience in front of the camera; and the shopping channel products are not limited to clothes or jewelry but also encompass every sort of food, including pizza crusts. However, media representations of food and eating have not always been popular in Japan.

Masahiro Shindo has analyzed the travel diaries of Japanese writers who visited Europe and Italy during the Meiji era (1868–1912) and the Taisho period (1912–1926).[19] He focused, in particular, on the culinary dimensions of the diaries, pointing out that food and eating descriptions were infrequent and inaccurate. Probably in the Meiji and Taisho periods, he speculates, the Japanese considered eating as a private activity that was not worth mentioning publicly. Or, perhaps, the Japanese palate was not used to foreign food and could not discern between good or not-so-good dishes. He did, however, find a few scattered references to food among the diary pages.

For instance, Toyotaka Komiya, apprentice to and biographer of Soseki Natsume, reported visiting the restaurant Umberto in Rome in January 1924 in his *Itaria Nikki* (Italian diary). At that time, it was assumed to be the best restaurant in town, but, although food descriptions are missing, Komiya reported that he did not enjoy his meal. In contrast, a few days later, on January 27, he visited Nemi Lake, and, on the way back to Rome, he stopped at a restaurant near the train station to have mixed fried fish and shrimp. This dish he did enjoy, because, as he wrote, it resembled Japanese tempura. During the following days, Komiya visited Naples and, in the entry dated February 1, he briefly described his dinner at a seafood restaurant. He had a fish soup, made with slices of sea bass and squid, tomatoes, and breadcrumbs. According to his writing, it was an excellent soup. As noted by Shindo, it appears that Komiya appreciated seafood and all the dishes that reminded him of Japanese cuisine. In fact, risotto was one more dish that appeared to be valued by Japanese travelers. It seems from these food notes that the intent was not to describe a different cuisine but to find some sort of affinity with Japanese cooking through similar or common ingredients or dishes such as fish, rice, and tempura.

References to food became slightly more common and accurate in the 1950s. For instance, the economist Shinzo Koizumi visited postwar Italy, and he reported in his diary entry on July 28, 1953,

> At 7:30 p.m., invited by the Ambassador and his wife, I am introduced to a small *trattoria* overlooking a petite square with a fountain (Piazza S. Maria in Trastevere). The eatery name is Galeazzi, and it is located in the Trastevere neighborhood at the end of a tiny street where cars can barely enter. Outside the premises there are about ten tables .... We hailed a man who looked like the head waiter. He took a random piece of paper and, using a pencil, he wrote down what follows:
>
> 1) Prosciutto e melone, 2) Cannelloni, 3) Grissine [sic], 4) Vino Soave.
>
> **1)** It is a starter, and prosciutto is hamu [ham] and melone is meron [melon]. The dish is dry-cured ham served alongside melon. It might seem like an unusual match, but I have been told it is quite popular in Italy.
>
> **2)** [Cannelloni] consist of white flour dough wrapped around minced meat. They are served with some broth on the top and sprinkled with grated cheese. It is a typical Italian dish.
>
> **3)** Grissini is a type of pencil-shaped bread.[20]

Cannelloni and *prosciutto e melone* as well as grissini are now popular fare in Japan. This is true not only in eateries specializing in Italian cuisine but also in many general family restaurants. The fact that Koizumi felt the need to explain the dishes shows that Italian cuisine was not very popular among the Japanese in the 1950s, not even among the wealthiest or educated.

In his anthropological study and memoir *Meeting with Japan*, Fosco Maraini wrote, "the French is the only European influence which is not restricted to the world of culture ... but has spread into everyday life." A few pages later we read, "the Japanese certainly know little about Italy, and what they know tends to come to them through writers of other countries."[21] This account, once again, testifies to the hegemonic role played by French culture at the time.

Indeed, things have changed since Koizumi encountered and described Italian food and Maraini reported about his knowledge of Italian culture in Japan. Slowly but surely, Italian culture and Italian products have managed to penetrate Japanese everyday life.

By the mid 1980s, upscale Tokyo businessmen were wearing expensive Giorgio Armani suits, and even trend-conscious Japanese gangsters switched from Lincolns and Mercedes-Benzes to Lamborghinis and Maseratis.[22] Moreover, it was no longer necessary to be well-off to have a taste of Italy. Family restaurants began to feature Italian dishes on their menus, and restaurants specializing in Italian cuisine became popular (e.g., Saizeriya, La Pausa, and Capricciosa).[23]

By the 1990s, popular magazines had begun promoting products that were all Italian and the Italian *ishokuju* (clothing, food, and housing). Along with Italian goods, Italian food acquired a special status among female consumers, who defined the food as *kigaru de yasui* (cheerful and inexpensive). In those years, the popular magazine *Hanako* favored the tiramisu and the panna cotta boom.[24] It may seem trivial, but, as pointed out by Katarzyna Cwiertka[25] and John Clammer,[26] booms are important in understanding the Japanese consumer culture. Sometimes trends are followed simply because it is difficult not to follow them. Shops fully invest in the current boom and stop carrying the stock reflecting the previous one. Trend awareness is a signal of social integration.[27] In the 1990s, the *itameshi* boom exploded onto the Japanese dining-out experience. The interest in Italian cuisine did not fade away but rather grew and, as a result, became more specialized. However, the seeds of the Italian cuisine had been planted many years before the *itameshi* boom.

As revealed in the travel diaries previously mentioned, Italian cuisine was basically unknown to Japanese. Nevertheless, between the 1940s and 1950s, Italian cuisine tiptoed into the Japanese scene due to the efforts of several Italian, American, and Japanese individuals. Among the pioneers of Italian cuisine in Japan, we should count the chefs and kitchen workers of an Italian military vessel that arrived in Kobe in 1943: Antonio Cancemi, Giuseppe Donnaloia, Orazio Abela and Luigi Fidanza each created legacies that still live on today. At the end of the war, they remained in Japan, where they continued their cooking careers. Cancemi started working in a small German restaurant in Kobe and served for a month as chef to General Douglas MacArthur on a train trip around Japan in 1946. Later, Cancemi moved his headquarters from Kobe to Tokyo where, in 1957, he opened the restaurant Antonio's, which is currently managed by his grandchildren.

Donnaloia opened his restaurant in Kobe in 1952. The original premises collapsed during the Great Hanshin-Awaji Earthquake in 1995; however, the restaurant Donnaloia is still in business. It is currently managed by a Japanese chef, Motori Watabe. In 1946, Abela opened Amore Abela in the area of Takarazuka. The restaurant is currently run by Abela's son, Ercole Abela. Fidanza did not open his own restaurant but became the head chef of Ristorante Hanada in Tokyo. During their careers, Cancemi, Donnaloia, Fidanza, and Abela trained many Japanese cooks.

An additional popular restaurant at the time was Nicola's Pizza House, which the Italian-American Nicola Zappetti opened in 1956. Zappetti was not a trained chef but was a marine who stayed in Japan after the war and found success serving Italian-American cuisine and pizza. During the same period, Takayasu Narimatsu opened Kabe no Ana (Hole in the Wall) in 1953. His restaurant specialized in Japanized versions of spaghetti. Kabe no Ana is now a popular restaurant chain with branches all over Japan and across Asia.

Before the 1960s, there were only a few Japanese chefs and restaurateurs who served traditional Italian cuisine. Among them, Haruko Horikawa is worth mentioning. In 1962, she ran the restaurant Carina, a small Italian eatery, located in the Isetan department store of Shinjuku. In 1968, she became the chef of the restaurant Toscana, contributing to the birth of Italian regional cuisines in Japan. Her interest in Italian cuisine began in 1932 when she moved to Rome and served as a maid at the Japanese embassy for the next five years.

The year 1964 was a landmark for the development of the Italian culinary scene in Japan. On April 1, 1964, Japanese restrictions on overseas travel were lifted. With the liberalization of overseas traveling, Europe became a viable destination for Japanese. Thus, those who went to Italy, whether they were simple tourists or chefs in training, now had the chance to discover Italian cuisine firsthand. For example, Toshiaki Yoshikawa, owner and chef of Ristorante Capitolino, moved to Italy in 1965, and Mamoru Kataoka, owner and chef of Ristorante al Porto, went to Italy in 1968. Yoshikawa and Honda received their training at the ENALC Hotel (Ente Nazionale Lavoratori del Commercio), a hotelier school near Rome that provided local and foreign chefs with working experience inside Italian hotels and restaurants.[28] During the peak of the *itameshi* boom, chefs who had received training in Italy were treasured by the dining market. Also, young cooks, who had been educated only at Japanese culinary schools, became increasingly interested in overseas apprenticeships. Overseas training became highly valued. For instance, the popular restaurant Acqua Pazza opened in 1990 employing only Italy-trained personnel. This accounts for the power of the training system that provided cooks with job skills as well as with cultural and social capital. It also shows the transitional nature of power pointed out by Gregory et al.[29] Japanese cooks moved from a status of power-receiving apprentices in Italy to a status of power-holding cooks and trainers in Japan.

Nobuo Nishimura must be mentioned among the influential contributors involved in establishing a training network between Italy and Japan. Although not a chef, he studied Italian language and culture at Tokyo University of Foreign Languages. He established Bunryu Co. Ltd., an association aimed at promoting cultural exchange between the two countries. He started by importing Italian books and publishing Italian-Japanese dictionaries. Later, he set up an Italian language school, which now has branches in Italy. In 1973, he founded the restaurant Bunryu. In order to promote authentic Italian cuisine, he signed training agreements with the ENALC Hotel, where he also organized a month-long course for Japanese chefs. When the ENALC closed, he was involved in the establishment of a culinary academy in Siena, in 1987, called La Scuola Internazionale di Cucina Italiana di Siena. Eventually, the Siena school closed with the retirement of its Italian founders, but a new branch opened in the nearby Tuscany city of Lucca and is still in operation today. Currently, Bunryu sends about twenty chef apprentices each year to the school in Lucca.

Among the notable training schools offering long-term as well as short-term courses to Japanese cooks and chefs are the Italian Culinary Institute for Foreigners (ICIF) and the Italian Culinary Tours (ICT), both located in Piedmont. ICIF, based in Costigliole D'Asti, first opened in 1991, and it welcomed its first group of Japanese students in 1992. Today, apprentices from many countries train there, but the majority remain Japanese. ICT is a culinary tour operator established in 1995. Among its services are cooking classes, dedicated only to Japanese apprentices, held at the Istituto Alberghiero Rosmini of Domodossola, a vocational high school specializing in hospitality.

Thus, the training of Japanese chefs in Italian cuisine followed a mixed and open path. Before the 1960s, culinary schools in Japan primarily offered French training. Many of the chefs interested in Italian cooking worked in the restaurants run by Italian pioneer chefs. They decided to improve their skills and gain firsthand experience by going to Italy. When these chefs returned to Japan and became successful, especially in the 1990s, they became the trainers of a new batch of Japanese apprentices interested in Italian cuisine, moving from being at the receiving end of power to being power holders. Meanwhile, culinary schools in Italy offered their services to the Japanese. It is important to point out that this Italian training system was an open system in which anyone willing to learn (and having the economic resources) was able to participate and gain experience. This open system and this transitional nature of power are particularly evident in the case of apprentice pizza makers (namely the *pizzaiolo*), as described in the following section.

The Napoli pizza and the *pizzaiolo*

In addition to the tiramisu and panna cotta booms of the 1990s, there was also the Napoli pizza boom, which was favored by the establishment of Italian pizzerias such as Da Salvatore and Savoy (1995), both located in the area of Naka Meguro. In September 1996, the lifestyle magazine *Brutus* invited three pizza masters from Naples, namely Raffaele Surace, Gaetano Fazio and Gaetano Esposito, to Japan. They were to test the state of pizza in the country. Italian *pizzaiolos* moved to Japan to ply their trade, and Japanese went to Italy, especially to Naples, to learn the art of crafting a traditional pizza. Some of them even joined Italian pizza associations. For instance, Akio Nishikawa earned coveted the VPN certification (Verace Pizza Napoletana, True Neapolitan Pizza) for his pizzeria Sakuragumi in Hyogo prefecture in 1997.

Over the following years, Japanese *pizzaiolos* made headlines by winning pizza competitions in Italy. Italian associations promoting original pizza napoletana established independent branches in Japan. The most popular among these is the Associazione Verace Pizza Napoletana (AVPN), which opened a Japanese office in 2006. Today, the group's membership numbers sixty-four certified pizzerias throughout Japan.[30] More recently, in 2012, the Associazione Pizzaiuoli Napoletani (APN) also established a local office, and it counts twenty pizzerias in its group.[31] In 2016, the Japanese press reported a second wave of the Napoli pizza boom.[32] This boom will probably be more intense than the first boom, which was part of the *itameshi* phenomenon. Italian and Japanese *pizziaolos* are often featured in magazines and television programs.

Japan is not famous for being a country of *pizzaiolos*, but their work is, nevertheless, recognized as a specialty occupation requiring skills taught at vocational and culinary schools. A website specializing in vocational schools in the Kansai area presents a description of the *pizzaiolo* as follows:

> Along with expert *boulangers* and professional bread makers, there is growing interest in artisans specializing in pizza. In the realm of Italian cuisine, the *cuoco* (chef) is a separate profession. The *pizzaiolo* has many responsibilities, which include monitoring and operating the oven, molding the dough, baking, and making one complete pizza. Moreover, the knowledge of different cuisines and various ingredients is becoming a requirement, and *pizzaiolos* are now attracting attention for their creativity and their original toppings. According to a pizza craftsman, it is by training and building experience, by learning the proper posture that the technique will be authentic. To become a first-class artisan, you have to use nothing else but your hands.[33]

The term *pizza shokunin* is used to indicate a pizza artisan, and the word ピッツァイオーロ (*pizzaiolo*) has entered the Japanese katakana dictionary.[34]

Needless to say, the occupation had its origin in Italy, specifically in Naples. *Pizzaiolo* schools have mushroomed all over Italy. They are organized by countless pizza associations to deal with the growing requests for *pizzaiolos* in Italy and abroad. *Pizzaiolo* courses are sometimes patronized and funded by the local Italian administration as a countermeasure against unemployment. However, the craft of pizza making is still, as a rule, learned through apprenticeships at a pizzeria. In traditional pizzerias, the roles (preparation duties) are typically carried out by three persons working around a wood oven in a hierarchical structure: at the head, is the *pizzaiolo*, who makes the dough, rolls it out, and prepares the topping; then a baker, who is in charge of baking the pizza; and finally, the table assistant, who is in charge of such tasks as slicing the mozzarella and placing the ingredients in their respective containers. However, the precise division of tasks is becoming less common as the assistants are now also involved in making pizza, and the apprenticeship time has been shortened. Usually, a *pizzaiolo* acquires skills at an early age, often continuing in a family tradition. The *pizzaiolo* is a sought-after figure in the restaurant business. Many Italian *pizzaiolos*, mainly from southern Italy, have experience working abroad, particularly in Europe and in the Americas. Since the late 1980s, Japan has appeared as a more exotic and lucrative destination for *pizzaiolos* seeking experience abroad.

Generally, when an Italian *pizzaiolo* arrives in Japan, he already has a job, some kind of accommodation, and a visa sponsorship. Contacts with Japanese restaurateurs and food companies are made in Italy through informal networks of friends and acquaintances working in the restaurant business. The network is built by participating in hospitality fairs, pizza events, and competitions around Italy as well as joining one of the above-mentioned pizza associations. Usually, the Italian *pizzaiolo* does not have strong knowledge of Japanese culture and does not speak the local language. Nevertheless, he has what it takes to ply his trade in Japan (i.e., working skills and cultural capital).

There are also *pizzaiolos* who are sent to Japan for a few months by Italian pizza chains entering the market (e.g., Rosso Pomodoro). They are in charge of supervising the opening of the shop abroad. Italian *pizzaiolos* are not only responsible for setting up the pizza menu but also for training the Japanese *pizzaiolos*. Afterward, they move to a new destination and a new kitchen.

However, the most successful Japanese *pizzaiolos* are those who have received their training in Italy. The majority went to Italy during the 1990s. Still, the possibility that some Japanese *pizzaiolos* traveled to Italy for this purpose before the 1990s cannot be ruled out. This is because, at that time, *pizzaiolos*, in contrast to chefs, were often not formally trained in culinary schools. Most men who want to be *pizzaiolos* go to Italy on tourist or student visas and search for on-the-spot training at a pizzeria. This informal condition of flux and the lack of official data make exact training times or starting points difficult to account for.

Pizzaiolos who first moved to Italy were at the receiving end of power, and they experienced difficulties in finding a place to work, in particular in finding an appropriate traditional apprenticeship. The *maestro pizzaiolo* judges and decides whether or not the apprentice might be allowed to enter the pizzeria and work around the oven. As one Japanese *pizzaiolo* who went to Naples in 1998 and spent a total of seven years in Italy reported,

> I ate in many pizzerias, and when I liked the place I asked: Can I work here? I wish to learn the cooking ways of this pizzeria. And some places told me it was not possible because I had no experience, but I decided I wanted to work for Gaetano Esposito because I really liked the pizza he made. But once he had told me he would not take Japanese guys, only Neapolitans. But then, when I went back the third time, he said, "You must really love my pizza." And then he gave me a one-week trial period. And then he said, "Ok, I will take you in." He told me I was different from other Japanese, the ones telling him that they wanted to learn, just to look . . . but I had told him I wanted to learn the job, I wanted to work. I was not looking for a school. Then I started working with him. And he has been nice; he taught me a lot of things.[35]

When a Japanese apprentice becomes acquainted with and forms a close relationship with his master and coworkers, there is a level of acceptance. He might even receive an Italian nickname. For instance, Akinari Makishima, a pizza competition winner in 2006 and 2010, is also known as Pasquale, named after his Italian pizza master. A nickname can also be chosen because the Japanese name sounds similar to the Italian (e.g., Yuiji becomes Luigi or Hichiro becomes Ciro). Once the young Japanese apprentice is accepted into a pizzeria, chances are he will then be introduced to other pizzerias and learn different methods.

When the apprenticeship period in Italy is over, the Japanese *pizzaiolo* returns to Japan with newly acquired job skills and cultural knowledge. He will have learned not only how to make pizza but also that there are different kinds of pizza and pizza tastes throughout Italy.

However, not every aspiring *pizzaiolo* has the chance to move to Italy. The encounter with pizza can take place casually in one of the many Italian restaurants of Tokyo. Young Japanese start working in the kitchen and then they move to the oven. The move from the kitchen to the oven can be considered a chance to distinguish oneself in the crowded world of Italian restaurants. In the words of a Japanese chef-restaurateur,

> Nowadays, pizza napoletana has become so popular, especially in Tokyo, that a lot of chefs are willing to become *pizzaiolos*. As a matter of fact, my boys, working in the kitchen or as hall staff, have the desire to make pizza. To me it is easy. I do not have to look for *pizzaiolos*; they come to me because they want to learn.[36]

The above statement bears witness to the power held by those who have received their training abroad and are highly valued as they can teach pizza making to the ones who did not go to Italy, even to the cooks who, in the hierarchy of the culinary profession, occupy a higher position.

While moving from the kitchen to the oven might look like a smooth passage, there are cases in which the Japanese *pizzaiolo* does not come from a culinary background. Others have become pizza chefs as a result of a general interest in pizza or Italy. For instance, Satoshi Ikuta, owner and *pizzaiolo* of the popular Roman-style pizzeria Il Pentito, used to work as a buyer for a fashion company when he decided, in 1988, at the age of thirty-six, to move to Rome and learn how to make pizza. Yasumasa Yoshikawa, manager of Pizzeria Dream Factory, shares a similar story. He was the third-generation owner of a laundry shop in Tokyo. However, he had been impressed by Italian pizza during a holiday in Florence and decided to become a *pizzaiolo*. He first received his training at a Tokyo pizza restaurant, and then he went to Italy to buy an oven and to receive a *pizzaiolo* certification. In 1994, he turned his laundry shop into a pizzeria.

These last two examples show that Japanese do not only go to Naples to learn pizza skills. In a further example, Takeshi Morita worked and received his training near the city of Ravenna for about three years. In 2001, he won the Gusto della Pizza (Taste of Pizza) prize in a competition held at the Padua Pizza Show.

Satoshi Ikuta and Yasumasa Yoshikawa are examples of Japanese entrepreneurs who opened their own pizzerias without any formal culinary training. However, they both had business and trade experience, and this probably accounts for the relative ease with which they ventured into opening successful restaurants.

In some cases, the Japanese *pizzaiolo* did not attend a culinary school and had little business or trade experience. For instance, Yoshihisa Otsubo, owner of the successful Pizzeria il Tamburello, graduated from college with a degree in European Philosophy. In 1994, he traveled to Europe. At that time, he had no interest in pizza or the possibility of becoming a *pizzaiolo*. One day, as he was walking along the streets of Naples, he was approached by a young Italian student majoring in Japanese. He invited Otsubo first to dinner at his place and then to share a pizza at one of the most famous pizzerias in town. Otsubo was, in turn, so impressed with this incident that he decided to learn how to make pizza. His new Italian friend introduced him to the owner of a pizzeria. In the following passage, he recalls his new part-time job,

> I asked to work. Even washing the dishes would be fine. So I worked only during the weekends, but this way I could also see the work of the *pizzaiolo* and what kind of job it was. It was fascinating: the atmosphere of the pizzeria, the laughing and the joke telling. The atmosphere of Italian

> restaurants in Japan was, how would you say, completely different.... Fourteen years ago Italian restaurants [in Japan] were like conservative French restaurants.[37]

These remarks testify again to the powerful role played by French cuisine and how it served as a role model for Italian restaurants. It also shows the multifaceted nature of power: a young man with a degree in philosophy asked to learn a manual job and started by washing the dishes. He is on the receiving end of power, but, at the same time, he is learning.

Thus, Japanese *pizzaiolos* come from various occupational and social backgrounds. Usually, they begin working in Italian restaurants as waiters or cooks and then decide to train to be a *pizzaiolo*. There are also cases in which the *pizzaiolo* lacks a culinary background but, nevertheless, decides to enter the occupation because of a personal interest in Italian culture and cuisine. Yet there are two main paths to becoming a high-status pizzaiolo: (i) looking for a restaurant job where the *pizzaiolo* is Italian or has been trained in Italy and (ii) traveling to Italy. Nowadays, given the growing links and networks between Italy and Japan regarding the pizza trade, most of the Japanese traveling to Italy have already arranged for pizzeria employment through connections. These connections had been established through the first Japanese who moved to Italy, the Italian *pizzaiolos* in Japan, and the Italian pizza associations now based in Japan.

Moreover, pizza courses are now featured at Japanese culinary and vocational schools. Still, as noted by both Italian and Japanese informants, the various courses can be considered a mere introduction to the art of making pizza, which can only be fully learned through working experience. Japanese *pizzaiolos* who have undertaken years of apprenticeships in Italy enjoy more respect within their occupational community. Furthermore, *pizzaiolos* who have participated in and won pizza competitions are more highly valued in the Japanese market. Winning pizza awards acquires institutionalized cultural capital: embodied cultural capital made tangible, legalized, and marketable through formal certifications.[38] A pizza award is a form of a cultural prize that can lead to a career promotion. The possession of such awards also easily opens the door to magazine and television appearances. The institutionalized cultural capital helps popularize Japanese *pizzaiolos* in and outside of the restaurant sphere.

Conclusions

The decade between 1985 and 1995 represented the golden age of Italian food in Japan. During the so-called *itameshi* boom, dining on Italian food—more or less authentic or Japanized—became fashionable. The popularity of

Italian cuisine continued to grow well beyond the boom. The market evolved to include the different regional cuisines, and the kitchen *campanilismo* is nowadays well represented in the Japanese dining scene. A diverse set of reasons explains the spread and popularity of the Italian cuisine that, over a relatively short period of time, has firmly established itself in modern Japanese culture. The most significant and previously mentioned reasons for this trend were the newly accessible opportunities to travel overseas, interest in products Made in Italy (e.g., fashion and furniture), and young women with newly acquired available income looking for a stylish and healthy, but not too expensive, cuisine.

However, we have focused our attention on the role played by culinary professionals who exert power in the production and distribution of Italian cuisine in Japan. In fact, going back to the definition of power given at the beginning of this chapter, we have stated that people experience power every day by exercising or receiving it, but more important than the fact that power is exercised is the way in which power is constructed and deployed.[39] The power of chefs and pizzaiolos has been constructed and organized via personal networks and a training system built over the years between Italy and Japan, connecting Italian and Japanese cooks as well as culinary associations and cooking schools at different levels.

As we have seen, before the mid-1980s, Italian cuisine was not widespread in Japan. It was a counterhegemonic cuisine. There were, however, some pioneer chefs whose restaurants served as schools for Japanese cooks. Some of the cooks from these kitchens traveled to Italy to receive overseas training and continue their apprenticeship abroad in restaurants and culinary schools. When they returned to their home country, particularly at the beginning of the 1990s, they found a market ready to receive Italian cuisine and that was looking for experts in the field. The Italian culinary scene had grown stronger and diversified itself, thereby creating new opportunities for *pizzaiolos*.

Similar to cooks, pizza makers moved to Italy to undertake a period of apprenticeship, thus building a transnational network of professional pizza makers. A measure of the significance of the network is, for instance, evident in the establishment of professional associations such as the Association of Italian Chefs of Japan and AVPN Japan. The development of Italian food events, such as the Napoli Pizza Fest in Japan, also attests to the network's significance. Moreover, the training network has promoted the successful establishment of an Italian cuisine that has not only moved from being a countercuisine to mainstream but has also prospered beyond the *itameshi* boom and expanded beyond Japanese borders with the establishment of Japanese-Italian premises in other Asian countries.

Notes

1 The romanization of Japanese words follows the Hepburn system.

2 Katarzyna J. Cwiertka, *Modern Japanese Cuisine: Food, Power and National Identity* (London: Reaktion, 2006), 13–17 and 42–9.

3 Unless otherwise stated, this chapter refers to restaurants in Tokyo.

4 Warren Belasco, *Appetite for Change: How the Counterculture Took On the Food Industry* (Ithaca: Cornell University Press, 2006), terms as countercuisine the movement that in 1960s America opposed mainstream industrial processed food. Over the years, the countercuisine movement itself became mainstream, as testified by the ever-growing popularity of farmers markets, farm shops, and global movements such as Slow Food. In a similar vein, French cuisine represented the hegemonic foreign cuisine in Japan, while Italian cuisine was a countercuisine that, nowadays, itself holds a hegemonic position.

5 Derek J. Gregory et al., *The Dictionary of Human Geography*, 5th ed. (Chichester, UK: Wiley-Blackwell, 2009), 575.

6 Pierre Bourdieu, "The Forms of Capital," in *Readings in Economic Sociology*, ed. Nicole Woolsey Biggart (Malden, MA: Blackwell Publishers, 1986), 280–91.

7 Ernesto De Martino and Clara Gallini, *La fine del mondo: contributo all'analisi delle apocalissi culturali* (Torino: Einaudi, 1977).

8 Fabio Parasecoli, *Al Dente: A History of Food in Italy* (London: Reaktion Books, 2014), 257.

9 Franco Mosino, "Vocabolario Etimologico della Pasta Italiana," *Accademia Barilla*, 2011, accessed May 15, 2016, http://storage.aicod.it/portale/academiabarilla/file/VOCABOLARIO_ETIMOLOGICO_DELLA_PASTA.pdf.

10 Vittorio Agnetti, *La nuova cucina delle specialità regionali: piemontesi, ligure, lombarde, venete, emiliane, romagnole, toscane, romane, napoletane, siciliane e sardegnole* (Milano: Società editoriale milanese, 1909), preface translated from the Italian.

11 Massimo Montanari and Beth Archer Brombert, *Italian Identity in the Kitchen, or Food and the Nation* (New York: Columbia University Press, 2013).

12 Franco La Cecla, *La pasta e la pizza* (Bologna: Il Mulino, 1998); Alberto Capatti and Massimo Montanari, *La Cucina italiana: storia di una cultura* (Roma: Laterza, 2005).

13 Parasecoli, *Al Dente, 226.*

14 Simone Cinotto, *The Italian American Table: Food, Family, and Community in New York City* (Chicago: University of Illinois Press, 2013).

15 Anne Reynolds, "A Short History of Italian Cafés and Restaurants in Sydney," *Modern Greek Studies (Australia and New Zealand)* 10 (2013): 136–55.

16 Olivier De Maret, "More than Just Getting By: Italian Food Businesses in Brussels at the Turn of the Twentieth Century," *Food and Foodways* 21 (2013): 108–31; Ulrike Thoms, "From Migrant Food to Lifestyle Cooking: The Career of Italian Cuisine in Europe," *European History On-Line*, June 21, 2011, accessed May 15, 2016, http://ieg-ego.eu/en/threads/europe-on-the-road/economic-migration/ulrike-thoms-from-migrant-food-to-lifestyle-cooking-the-career-of-italian-cuisine-in-europe; Maren Möhring, "Staging and Consuming the Italian Lifestyle. The Gelateria and the Pizzeria-Ristorante in Post-war Germany," *Food and History* 7 (2009): 181–202.

17 Thoms, "From Migrant Food."

18 Data retrieved from the Ministry of Internal Affairs and Communications, Statistics Bureau, accessed May 30, 2016, http://www.stat.go.jp/.

19 Masahiro Shindo, "Semiologia della Letteratura Gourmet: Italia Vista, Mangiata e Bevuta dai Giapponesi," in *Nuove Prospettive di Ricerca sul Giappone*, ed. Giorgio Amitrano and Silvana De Maio (Napoli: Aistugia, 2012), 1–17.

20 As reported in Shindo, "Semiologia della Letteratura Gourmet," 12.

21 Fosco Maraini and Eric Mosbacher, *Meeting with Japan* (New York: Viking Press, 1959), 178 and 181.

22 Joseph J. Tobin, *Re-made in Japan: Everyday Life and Consumer Taste in a Changing Society* (New Haven, CT: Yale University Press, 1992), 37–41.

23 Indeed, family restaurants have played an important role in popularizing Italian cuisine, especially vis-à-vis French cuisine. As a rule, family and fast food restaurants arrived primarily during the 1970s in Japan via the United States (e.g., McDonald's, Denny's, KFC). The family restaurant market diversified, serving a mix of international and Japanese food (e.g., Royal Host), Japanese dishes (e.g., Otoya), or Asian cuisine (e.g., Bamiyan). In the family restaurant scene, Italian cuisine has proliferated. There are no French equivalents of Saizeriya. French cuisine has always been considered to be too formal. For instance, it is often included on the menu for traditional Japanese weddings at the Meiji Shrine of Tokyo (Ofra Goldstein-Gidoni, "The Making and Marking of 'Japanese' and the 'Western' in Japanese Contemporary Material Culture," *Journal of Material Culture* 6 [2001]: 67–90). Thus, we can speculate that it does not seem to fit into the family restaurant atmosphere.

24 Merry I. White, "Ladies Who Lunch: Young Women and the Domestic Fallacy in Japan," in *Asian Food: the Global and the Local*, ed. Katarzyna J. Cwiertka and Boudewijn C. Walraven (Honolulu: University of Hawaii Press, 2001), 63–75 and Merry I. White, "All Roads Lead to Home: Japanese Culinary Tourism in Italy," in *Japanese Tourism and Travel Culture*, ed. Sylvie Guichard-Anguis and Okpyo Moon (London: Routledge, 2009), 203–13; Toshio Miyake, "Italian Transnational Spaces in Japan: Doing Racialised, Gendered and Sexualised Occidentalism," *Cultural Studies Review*, 19 (2013): 100–24.

25 Cwiertka, *Modern Japanese Cuisine.*

26 John Clammer, *Contemporary Urban Japan: A Sociology of Consumption* (Oxford, UK: Blackwell Publishers, 1997).

27 Clammer, *Contemporary Urban Japan*, 40–1.

28 The ENALC Hotel (Ente Nazionale Lavoratori del Commercio) was active between 1959 and 1975. The school opened again in 2014.

29 Gregory et al., *Dictionary*.

30 Associazione Verace Pizza Napoletana in Japan, http://japan.pizzanapoletana.org/pizzerie.php, accessed May 31, 2016.

31 Associazione Pizzaiuoli Napoletani in Japan http://www.pizzaiuolinapoletani.jp, accessed May 31, 2016.

32 Gendai Business http://gendai.ismedia.jp/articles/-/39689, accessed May 31, 2016.

33 Osaka Professional Training Colleges Association http://www.senmongakkou.info/dream_work/details.php?jid=297, accessed May 31, 2016; translated from Japanese.

34 *Sanseido's Concise Dictionary of Katakana Words* (Tokyo: Sanseido, 2005), 865.

35 Ceccarini interview with Yuichi Teratoko, Tokyo, April 28, 2009.

36 Ceccarini interview with Yoichi Watanabe, Tokyo, April 1, 2009.

37 Ceccarini interview with Yoshihisa Otsubo, Tokyo, July 26, 2008.

38 Bourdieu, "Forms of Capital."

39 Gregory et al., *Dictionary*.

PART TWO

Anthropological situations

When he buys an item of food, consumes it, or serves it, modern man does not manipulate a simple object in a purely transitive fashion; this item of food sums up and transmits a situation; it constitutes an information; it signifies.

ROLAND BARTHES, 1961

3

Waiters, writers, and power: From dining room commanders to the emotional proletariat

Christoph Ribbat

Agency and the "factotum"

Ernest Hemingway's "A Clean, Well-Lighted Place" may be the most well-known waiter story in the English language. One waiter serves brandy to a late guest who will not leave. The other puts up the shutters and turns off the lights. Stereotypical Hemingway heroes are off fishing trout, watching bull fights, and hunting game. Things are much different, though, in this 1933 piece of fiction. The older waiter states that he is "reluctant" to close the place at night "because there may be some one who needs the café."[1] Then the story elevates this waiter to a philosopher. We plunge into his stream of consciousness: his thoughts on how "it was all a nothing and a man was a nothing too," and the world "was nada y pues nada y nada y pues nada."[2] The old waiter takes on a powerful position in this story. A supposedly simple service worker turns into a nihilist thinker explaining the world.

Hemingway's story imagines a figure oscillating between acts of service and individual agency. It makes a very significant point: about real waiters, too. By definition, they wait to receive orders. In 1898, a waiter's manual warned its readers not to "assume or show too much authority over a guest."[3] As Joanne Finkelstein notes, the individual server may seem like a "factotum" even to twenty-first-century customers, his labor "purchased along with the meal."[4] Sociologists of the service society count restaurant staff among the members of the "emotional proletariat." Working in "front-line service jobs," they operate under "very explicit instructions concerning what to say and how to act."[5] At the same time, wait staff can also be seen as "directors of a theatrical performance." In culinary spaces, they shape customer expectations and their enjoyment of food, drinks, and sociality. Various "contests for power and privilege" are going on in restaurants. Waiters play central roles in them—and not always subservient ones.[6]

In order to learn more about the intellectual history of waiters, we need to explore the stories told about them. Plenty of these circulate, including the omnipresent "waiter there's a fly in my soup" jokes. It is a given that restaurant customers observe servers. They evaluate their performance, first emotionally and intellectually, and then, in most Western cultures, as they are considering tips. We should assume that writers and scholars make particularly complex observations about servers and their distinct social and cultural contexts. In their interpretations and stories—the fictional ones and those we are used to calling true—the waiter, like Hemingway's aging hero, appears as a figure shifting between servility and authority. He helps us understand questions of power and agency in the culinary world.

That said, there are not too many stories like "A Clean, Well-Lighted Place." Journalists, historians, and sociologists do not seem to pay much attention to waiters. If they do, they see them in much more critical terms than Hemingway did. Twentieth-century intellectuals George Orwell and Jean-Paul Sartre treat them as embodiments of inauthenticity and false consciousness. The waitress's case is different. But the relationship between male waiters and their intellectual observers has always bordered on the dysfunctional.[7]

This is surprising. After all, culinary figures moved into the public spotlight a few decades ago, thanks to the restaurant's rise as an everyday institution and the concomitant swelling of the food discourse. Celebrity chefs now count as autonomous artists (think Ferran Adrià or Grant Achatz) or as social reformers (think Jamie Oliver or Alice Waters). Once known only to faithful newspaper readers, restaurant critics have turned into food writers and media entrepreneurs.[8] Unlikely figures also get their share of attention. Growing the tomatoes that the New York City restaurant scene found particularly tasty, a small-time farmer named Tim Starks turned into a minor celebrity of the early twenty-first century, with his own book deal for a tomato memoir to boot.[9] More and more sociologists, anthropologists, historians, and literary critics are turning toward culinary questions, studying groups and individuals whose lives revolve around food and service. Against this background, it is striking how little we still know about waiters—as directors of restaurant performances or as members of the emotional proletariat.

In the shadow of the waitress

It is the waitress whose public visibility ranks up there with the most familiar figures of the food revolution. Women servers have inspired numerous authors, sociologists, historians, and journalists. Observing female employees in dining rooms, coffee shops, and restaurants, these authors foreground the interaction between oppression and objectification on the one hand and women's subversive agency on the other.

The first major sociological study in the field, Frances Donovan's *The Woman Who Waits* (1920) portrays the waitresses of early twentieth-century Chicago as members of the urban underclass. Donovan's heroines lead precarious lives. They encounter sexual objectification and hierarchical workplaces that assign the lowest positions to women servers. But Donovan also sketches waitresses as strong, independent, bohemian figures. She shows how they carve out niches for themselves, according to their own needs and desires. "Her life," Donovan notes about the "type" she investigates, "is spent in trying to escape definitions and to avoid suppressions."[10] Also set in Chicago's culinary world, the most important restaurant study of the mid-twentieth century develops a similar narrative. Sociologist William Foote Whyte's *Human Relations in the Restaurant Industry* devotes numerous pages to the "crying spells" of waitresses. Then again, Whyte notes that service employees use their crying "as a weapon to get attention and sympathy and to escape blame"[11]—and that the women employ numerous other, more assertive, everyday tactics to change their environment.[12] In a similar mode, Greta Foff Paules's 1990s study of New Jersey waitresses concentrates on the ways in which her protagonists "resist the symbolism of service." The waitress "is not a servant," Paules concludes, "but an independent businessperson or a soldier."[13]

Twentieth-century literary accounts of waitresses also concentrate on the tension between servility and agency. James Cain's 1941 noir novel *Mildred Pierce* treats waitressing as a key step in the protagonist's rise from suburban isolation to financial and personal independence. Raymond Carver's 1973 short story "They're Not Your Husband" portrays the employee of a diner as the object of the male gaze—eventually, though, she controls the emotional game. In a book published a year after Carver's story, America's chief oral historian found himself drawn to the waitress as well. Studs Terkel's 1974 *Working* presents the restaurant employee Dolores Dante as an eloquent, strong-minded thinker emphasizing her own agency. "I can't be servile," Dante states. "I give service. There's a difference."[14] Alison Owings's 2004 oral history *Hey Waitress! The USA from the Other Side of the Tray*, a key work on female servers, treats its heroines as the "chroniclers and commentators of our time."[15] In several recent coffee-table books, women servers are praised in images and texts. Authors and photographers construct the waitress as an eloquent example of female agency and blue-collar (though we should say pink-collar) confidence.[16]

The waitress, then, is a cultural heroine, not an "unsung" one. Why not the waiter? Numbers alone do not explain his absence from this discourse (though there are three waitresses to every waiter in the United States).[17] The symbolic realm offers more important reasons. American waitresses and waiters represent opposite ends of the culinary spectrum. The male server has always been associated with formality and aloofness. In the early twentieth century, the formative years of the middle-class restaurant, male waiters "evoked an aristocratic past," as historian Andrew Haley states.[18] Informal places employed women. Their presence promised "quick yet personable service."[19] In contrast, male servers were frequently seen as obstacles to the democratization of the restaurant experience. Their "scornful look" reinforced anxieties about whether the new clientele would belong.[20] And so, writers and sociologists interested in the agency of the powerless focus on women servers. In dining spaces, their work can be observed from up close. Observers easily grasp (or so they assume) the pressures from supervisors and customers and the processes of objectification. They follow the waitresses' actions, sometimes strategic, sometimes spontaneous, to acquire agency in this clearly defined world. Far less frequently objectified and seemingly closer to the powerful than to the disempowered, the waiter does not strike a comparable figure. "Waiters, believe me, have it easier," oral historian Owings explains, citing "the sexual implications" of service labor.[21] As Leon Elder notes, male wait staff seem "impersonal, detached, efficient, and not to be bantered with."[22] Aiming to find agency in the powerless, writers shy away from waiters. However tentative and performative the male servers' ties to the elite may be, they do obstruct the documentarist's interest in the common man—or woman.

The gendered character of service work further complicates the relationship between waiters and their observers. Hegemonically masculine military codes shaped the occupation in the nineteenth century. And yet, waiters have always performed emotional labor, a field traditionally coded as women's work.[23] Trying to please customers, they constantly interact with them in words and body language. In her classic study *The Managed Heart*, Arlie Hochschild argues that men who do emotional labor well "have slightly less in common with other men than women who do it well have with other women."[24] British sociologist Darren Nixon observes how contemporary working-class men tend to reject the interactions of service work. Nixon interprets this as a "defensive reaction to the increasingly aesthetic consumerized service economy."[25]

Writers and scholars may feel less threatened than Nixon's informants. But they also tend to shy away from these atypical service workers. Exploring masculinities of the past, labor historians foreground manual work, employees' resistance to power, and the practices of homosocial communities. As a result they pay less attention to protagonists heavily dependent on tips and active in the heterogeneous world of the restaurant.[26] As Ronnie Steinberg and Deborah Figart point out, gender conventions have led scholars in the field of emotional labor to "privilege" the exploration of women and to pay little attention to men performing similar jobs.[27]

There is a lot to be missed. Service workers, male and female, are always part of "cultural and aesthetic displays."[28] Within these displays, predetermined rules govern the way they express their emotions.[29] To "demonstrate concern for total customer satisfaction," the handbook of an early twenty-first-century gourmet deli asserts, in language characteristic of most culinary work places, that it is "each and every employee's" duty to mask their "troubles … with a smile." Rules like these are written for women and men both. However, it is the very notion of labor as masked performance that complicates the male waiter's identity. In Western modernity, masquerading has always been perceived as a feminine act. Male performances in everyday contexts thus irritate gender conventions.[30] And it is this complicated position that makes waiters particularly interesting. To move the focus toward them and away from waitresses should not be misunderstood as a revisionist project aiming to marginalize feminist studies of emotional labor. Instead, the male waiter's intellectual history opens another window on the way we think and write about service, power, and agency.

Orwell, Sartre, and the age of the open kitchen

In the literary history of restaurant work, Orwell's 1933 *Down and Out in Paris and London* ranks as a canonical text. The account explores the interwar years when throngs of expatriates frequented Parisian restaurants, cafes, and hotels—as consumers.[31] Orwell changed roles. As a kitchen laborer, he worked in a luxurious hotel and in a sophisticated restaurant. Recounting his experiences, he argues that luxury and sophistication are but very fine layers of pretense. A *plongeur*, the lowest figure in the French restaurant world, Orwell experienced extremely hard work, the dirt, and the rats behind the scenes; the steep hierarchies; and the back-breaking exploitation endemic to what is now known as the hospitality industry. Clearly, *Down and Out in Paris and London* takes sides. Orwell produced a hybrid of the slumming adventure story and the political essay. He opened the celebrated city of hotels and restaurants to a leftist critique of privilege and power. His narrative is part of a much larger tradition, the key agents of which historian Mark Pittenger, with a nod to Orwell, calls the "down-and-outers": middle-class observers claiming "a unique authority to speak of and for the poor."[32]

And yet, one type of restaurant worker does not seem to deserve the writer's working-class solidarity. The waiter's "skill," as Orwell states, "is chiefly in being servile." He is a "snob." He seems corrupted because he "lives perpetually in sight of rich people." He "sucks up to them with smiles and discreet little jokes." To "never be sorry for a waiter," Orwell declares, was the "moral" of his behind-the-scenes account. In contrast to cooks, the servers do not seem "workmanlike." In contrast to the ordinary kitchen help, they do not have pride. Orwell presumes (erroneously) that waiters do not form unions. They work extremely long hours, he notes, because "they find the servile nature of their work rather congenial."[33] Orwell and his fellow *plongeurs* are fending off exploitation and poverty. The waiters provide a counterpoint to their struggle.

Orwell's subsequent nonfiction project makes his dislike of waiters appear in even starker relief. Four years after *Down and Out in Paris and London*, Orwell published *The Road to Wigan Pier*, a portrait of British miners and a more wide-ranging reflection of class issues. Among these workers, Orwell finds more than just poverty. Exploring the potential of power among the powerless, he emphasizes their heroism and his own admiration for working-class identities. Going down to the mines with his protagonists, Orwell points out "what splendid men they are." It is a judgment based on their "most noble bodies." These Orwell describes in detail: "wide shoulders tapering to slender supple waists, and small pronounced buttocks and sinewy thighs, with not an ounce of waste flesh anywhere."[34] Miners' work appears as authentic and utterly significant in *The Road to Wigan Pier*. It is labor requiring enormous skill. "The miner's job," Orwell concludes, "would be as much beyond my power as it would be to perform on the flying trapeze or to win the Grand National."[35] This is work the world depends on. "Practically everything we do," Orwell notes, "from eating an ice to crossing the Atlantic, and from baking a loaf to writing a novel, involves the use of coal."[36]

In contrast, the body of the waiter as portrayed in *Down and Out in Paris and London* seems cartoonish rather than "splendid." Orwell describes how a server moves from the hidden part of the dining room into the area observed by guests: "The set of his shoulders alters; all the dirt and hurry and irritation have dropped off in an instant. He glides over the carpet with a solemn priest-like air."[37] The pretense certainly does not appear as labor, emotional or otherwise. It is just that, pretense. Whereas the miner's body and skills have the power to make the world turn, the waiter's performances lead Orwell to challenge the "real need of big hotels and smart restaurants."[38] This sort of work, he argues, produces "the shams that are supposed to represent luxury."[39] The waiter's transformations are integral parts of the system of "shams." This is what Orwell concludes—what he ignores, quite obviously, are the hotel's internal power structures regulating the waiter's practices.

Orwell's contemporaries did not necessarily share his hostility toward servers. In 1937, British waiter Dave Marlowe published *Coming, Sir!*, a memoir chronicling his adventures ranging from American speakeasies to transatlantic liners. Desmond MacCarthy contributed an introduction to Marlowe's work, marveling at "the screen of their polite alacrity standing between the server and the customers"[40] and praising waiters as "shrewd judges of human nature."[41] In Orwell's literary project, there is no admiration for "polite alacrity." Intensity, authenticity, and sincerity are the values Orwell evokes as his 1930s prose envisions a revolutionary power struggle in England. At the conclusion of *The Road to Wigan Pier* he imagines the middle classes joining forces with the working class in a "real Socialist party."[42] This kind of classlessness he reserves for those who do not serve the elite. Their dining room performances disconnect waiters from the power struggles of their time and from the agency Orwell associates with the working class.

When Sartre, another Orwell contemporary, examined the Parisian waiter, existential questions were more important than the revolutionary impulse. The server appears most prominently in *Being and Nothingness*, the philosopher's key work published in 1943 (an English translation appeared in 1956). In these passages, Sartre invites readers to reflect on "this waiter in the café." Like Orwell commenting on the service worker's "solemn, priest-like air," Sartre explores—and caricatures—body language first. He describes the specific waiter's movement as "quick and forward, a little too precise, a little too rapid," his "step a little too quick." The waiter "bends forward a little too eagerly." And "his voice, his eyes express an interest a little too solicitous for the order of the client." In the overall performance of the waiter, Sartre finds "the inflexible stiffness of some kind of automaton." He concludes, "We need not watch long before we can explain it: he is playing at being a waiter in a café."[43]

These passages appear in the second chapter of Sartre's *Being and Nothingness*, a segment devoted to the concept called "bad faith" (*mauvaise foi*). Whoever "practices bad faith," the philosopher explains, is lying to himself, "hiding a displeasing truth or presenting as truth a pleasing untruth."[44] Simplifying Sartre, the attitude of "bad faith" could be defined as a mode of thinking that is fundamentally different from "the responsible freedom of Being-for-itself," a central concept and goal of existential philosophy. People whose minds are dominated by bad faith confuse transcendence and facticity.[45] The waiter serves, in the café and on the page, as Sartre's example. Too eagerly performing on the job, he fails to distinguish between his real gestures and the gestures that are part of a server's performance. This makes "responsible freedom" impossible. Instead, Sartre's waiter finds himself in a situation similar to the one Orwell observed. Constantly playacting, he is disassociated from reality and, to follow Orwell's thoughts on the working class, from a world where bodies are as powerfully present as class identities.

Being and Nothingness is rich in ambiguities. So is Sartre's reading of the waiter. Following D. Z. Phillips's interpretation, we can only speculate on the meaning of "bad faith." Nor is it fully clear whether the waiter's performance marks him as an exceptionally alienated individual or, quite simply, as a human being. Sartre notes, though in a double negative, "It is by no means that [the waiter] can not form reflective judgments or concepts concerning his condition."[46] Certainly, we need to read Sartre's reflections on performance and "bad faith" in the context of their time, as indirect negotiations with Nazi Germany's ideology and performances military and political. And they are certainly more nuanced than Orwell's waiterphobic polemic. Nonetheless, the very complexity of Sartre's philosophical essay makes one unequivocal point: there is a significant difference between writer and waiter. In Hemingway's "A Clean, Well-Lighted Place," a service worker turns into a philosopher as the narrative voice pulls back to let the waiter's interior monologue take over. Agency emerges in bold relief—as the ability and authority to explain the world in the same way writers do. This certainly does not happen in Sartre's prose. Roles are clearly defined. As a philosopher, the author of *Being and Nothingness* consciously displays his own thinking as more complex and more attentive than anything emerging from the waiter's robotic mind.

A case in point: when Sartre describes a café in another chapter of *Being and Nothingness*, "with its patrons, its mirrors, its light, its smoky atmosphere, and the sounds of voices, rattling saucers, and footsteps which fill it," he attempts to explore the "fullness of being" found in the space.[47] Would the "automaton" waiter be able to do this? Probably not. And in the following pages, the author of *Being and Nothingness* latches his philosophical reflections to these descriptive segments. A discussion ensues about the concept of negation, triggered by Sartre's unsuccessful search for a friend expected to be present in the café. The philosopher is unable to find him. Thus, "what is offered to intuition is a flickering of nothingness."[48] The waiter, in contrast, revolves entirely around his own identity—as waiter. Nothingness does not flicker in his intuition. Rather, nothing much flickers at all. His "reflective judgments" are too simple. As Sartre speculates, they concern "the obligation of getting up at five o'clock, of sweeping the floor ... before the restaurant opens, of starting the coffee pot going"—or, perhaps, "the right to the tips, the right to belong to a union, etc."[49] According to Sartre, there is not much more the waiter has to offer to the world, certainly no monumental essay on phenomenological ontology.

Larger cultural patterns appear behind Orwell's and Sartre's thoughts. Orwell's distaste for the waiter is tightly linked to an antimodernist impulse emphasizing the significance of manual skills, in turn devaluing service work and emotional labor. This served a political function in the 1930s, particularly in Orwell's critique of totalitarianism from a working-class perspective. Reading Orwell his antipathy toward waiters as constantly performing snobs and his admiration for powerful miners reveal hegemonic notions of skill based on craftsmanship and manufacturing. As feminist scholars have argued, these concepts are heavily gendered. According to Steinberg and Figart, the "unacknowledged and uncompensated skills" of emotional labor are often women's skills.[50] As the male waiter's twentieth-century story shows, more issues are involved, and they include working-class myths and concepts of masculinity that are still latent today and that eclipse the public recognition of service work in general.

Sartre's insistence on autonomy and authenticity also reverberates in the foodie discourses of our time. However complex the reasoning in *Being and Nothingness*, popularized existentialism shaped postwar US culture. The reception of Sartre and Albert Camus connected to an American tradition of "the lonely individual" ready, as George Cotkin puts it, "to rebel against entrenched authority."[51] As Grace Hale's work demonstrates, existentialist concepts contributed to the larger transformation of American culture as a "nation of outsiders." Fictions of the authentic rebel became elements of a central narrative, writes Hale, "enabl[ing] Americans with political and economic power to disavow that power." Today, the "romance of the outsider," an imaginary figure alienated from social and cultural connections, influences American culture.[52] And to disavow power by emphasizing expressive, purportedly authentic individualism constitutes a central trait of twenty-first-century foodie culture.

Seventy years after Orwell and Sartre, the culinary elites have redefined how snobbery is performed. In contemporary restaurants, chefs are valued for the "freedom, professional virtuosity, originality, or authenticity" they represent. The performance of privilege does not seem to count anymore. Instead, the "subculturally authentic" seems particularly valuable, "smart casual," as food critic Alison Pearlman calls it.[53] Joseé Johnston and Shyon Baumann show how authenticity has emerged as "a key element of how foodies evaluate and legitimate food choices."[54] A fiction of classlessness dominates. Foodie discourse, Johnston and Baumann note, frequently depicts "impoverished people and locales as producing food that is all the more delicious for its connection to poverty."[55] Hierarchies, social and economic, seem to evaporate. So Sartre's robotic waiter appears as an uncomfortable reminder of the status and power imbalances hidden behind the new foodie aesthetics.

Chef's Story, a 2007 foodie coffee-table book, posits that contemporary chefs "are as nuanced as any artist, as business minded as any entrepreneur, and as hardworking as any coal miner."[56] Orwell's most admired laborers reemerge here. Service, though, the waiter's calling, is conspicuously absent. To think of the chef as a combination of artist, businessman, and blue-collar hero once again underscores his status as an autonomous and authentic individual. This combination now produces in contemporary culinary spaces what Pearlman calls "the theater of manual labor."[57]

Reflecting the public's desire to interact with chefs, the gourmet open kitchen epitomizes the dining room of the future. Customers observe sautéing chefs and cooks. As Pearlman notes, this is "theater," because there will always be a level of performativity to any action produced for the eyes of others. And it is theater with a backstage. More unattractive kinds of manual labor take place in invisible prep kitchens. These basement workspaces are as large as the actual restaurants themselves. And they send up their products to the kitchen before customers actually get to see them.[58] So the rearranged dining rooms hide two sorts of labor—prep work and service work. Their explicitly casual styles redefine the signifiers of social and economic inequality. They direct attention to those figures seen as powerful, creative, business minded, and physically forceful—the chefs—and away from the servers' performances categorized as inauthentic by leading twentieth-century intellectuals. In this new food culture, the waiter moves around in the shadows. To study his complexities, we need to turn away from the open kitchens and toward his long history.

In command: African American waiters, 1904

In 1859, Thomas A. Morris was born into slavery. The place was a town in the southern Appalachian Mountains, Sugar Hill, McDowell County, North Carolina. In the Reconstruction Era, Morris started working as a waiter at the Mountain Hotel in nearby Morganton. Even by late nineteenth-century standards, the place used an old-fashioned system. Instead of providing written menus, the cook would simply tell the service staff what the kitchen had to offer on a given day. In turn, the waiters informed the customers. Servers did not wear uniforms. Anything "neat and clean" sufficed. Morris soon moved on. He waited tables in other North Carolina and Kentucky

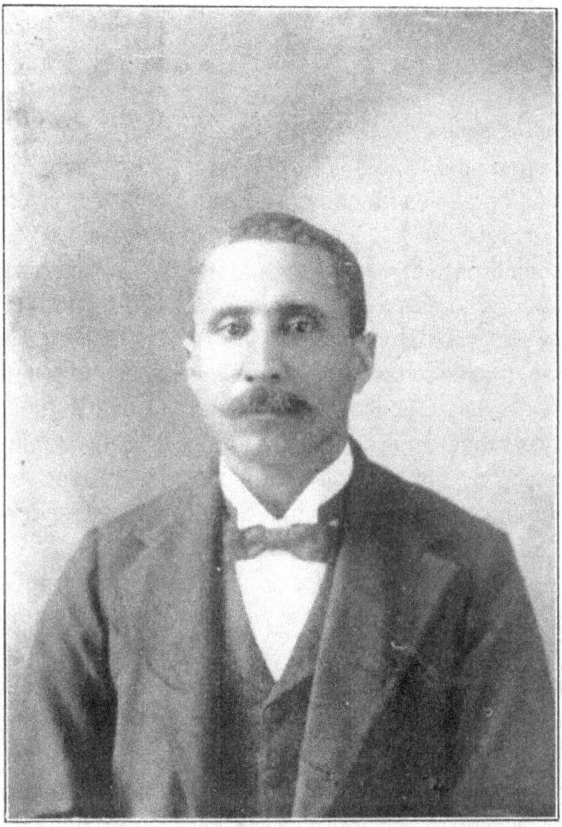

THOMAS A. MORRIS,

Headwaiter, Battery Park Hotel, Asheville, N. C.

FIGURE 3.1 *Thomas A. Morris. Headwaiter, Battery Park Hotel, Asheville, NC. From E. A. Maccannon,* Commanders of the Dining Room *(New York: Gwendolyn, 1904), 42.*

establishments. Finally he found an attractive long-term position at the Battery Park Hotel, an exclusive establishment in Asheville, North Carolina. In 1904, now forty-five years old, he posed for a photographer's camera. A comparatively powerful man, a headwaiter overseeing the Battery Park Hotel's dining room staff, Morris identified the modest Mountain Hotel, the place where he had started out, as most significant for his career.[59]

Morris's story can be found in a book titled *Commanders of the Dining Room: Biographic Sketches and Portraits of Successful Head Waiters*. In 1904, it was published under the auspices of an African American labor organization called the Head, Second and Side Waiters' National Benefit Association. Morris's story is one of fifty-two biographies collected in the book. All of them document the lives of black waiters. The author, E. A. Maccannon, is presumed to have been a waiter himself. The Library of Congress listed him as an African American writer.[60] *The Waiters, Hotel Bellmen and Railroad Porters' Journal* advertised in the opening pages of the book. So did one Hotel Champlain, claiming the "finest golf links in the Adirondacks."[61]

In the short biographies he composes and the waiters' words he quotes, Maccannon stresses an obvious detail that Orwell and Sartre ignore. Constantly moving between servility and agency, waiters shape their own stories. The men who seem like automatons to Sartre turn into individuals in *Commanders of the Dining Room*. The book tells of their lives in brief chapters. Often, these stories take us from the late nineteenth-century South to the North. One waiter, E. C. Holland, left Virginia and settled in Zanesville, Ohio. Raised in antebellum South Carolina, one Thomas J. Simons went off to work in New York City. A server named C. C. Randolph, born in Virginia "under the humid pressure of an adverse and humiliating social condition" (i.e., slavery), pursued his career in Massachusetts, New York, New Jersey, and finally took on a head waiter position in Edgemere, Long Island.[62] Using the circuits of the culinary world to move north, the waiters presented here preceded millions of fellow African Americans. The beginnings of the Great Migration from the segregated South to the North are usually thought to have begun in World War I. Historians evaluate the mass movement of individuals and families as a collective attempt to achieve, writes the historian Steven Reich, "economic and political freedom."[63] The African American waiters portrayed by Maccannon acquired this kind of freedom decades sooner.

In contrast to many of his colleagues, Thomas A. Morris remained in the South. This may explain why his reflections on servility and agency are particularly nuanced. Exploring his philosophy as headwaiter, Morris, the son of slaves, emphasizes his "policy" to "receive and obey orders"—terms that make his service work resemble the performances of servility associated with the slave system. And yet, when Morris notes that his "time and services" belonged to his employer the "entire time I was on duty," this clearly implies that they do not belong to the employer when he is not "on duty." Furthermore, he expresses the willingness to "execute an order promptly with little or no friction." This underscores his devotion to service. It also points at the explicit possibility of "friction" between waiter and employer, a concept taboo in the slave or Jim Crow system. Just as forcefully, Morris's life illustrates his agency. Throughout his waiting career, Morris moved from hotel to hotel, choosing his career options and ending up holding the coveted headwaiter position, achieved in his own independent negotiations on the

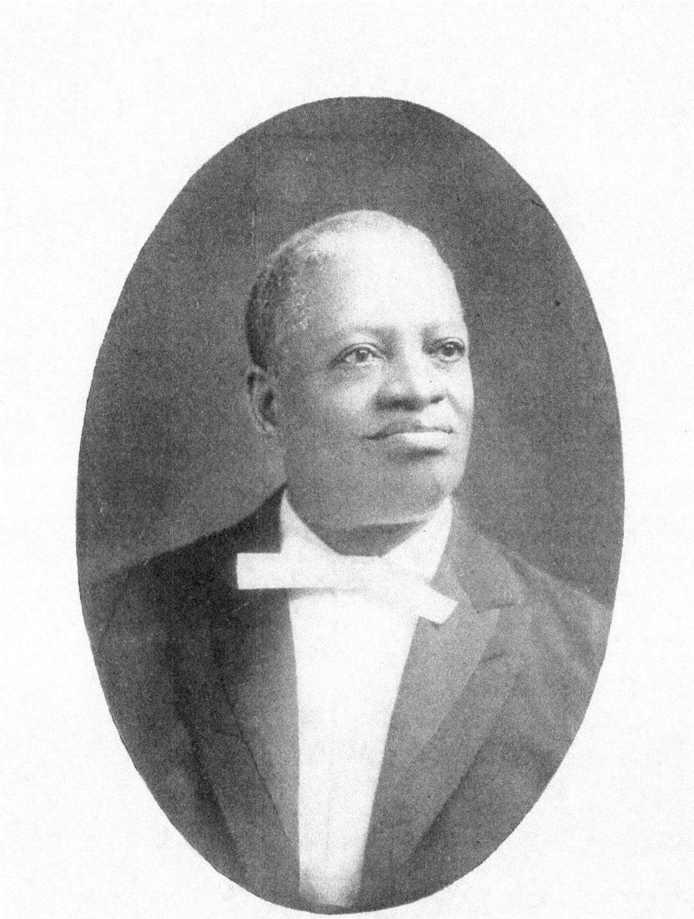

FIGURE 3.2 *Robert H. Grant. Headwaiter, McLure House, Wheeling, W. VA. From E. A. Maccannon,* Commanders of the Dining Room *(New York: Gwendolyn, 1904), 38.*

labor market. His skills "attract attention and bring their merited reward," Maccannon concludes—noting that future generations of African Americans, enjoying "a more fertile field and a freer atmosphere," would attain higher achievements.[64]

To white patrons of late nineteenth-century hotel dining rooms and upscale restaurants, the racialized dimensions of service must have seemed unequivocal. They were mostly waited on by African American men. This

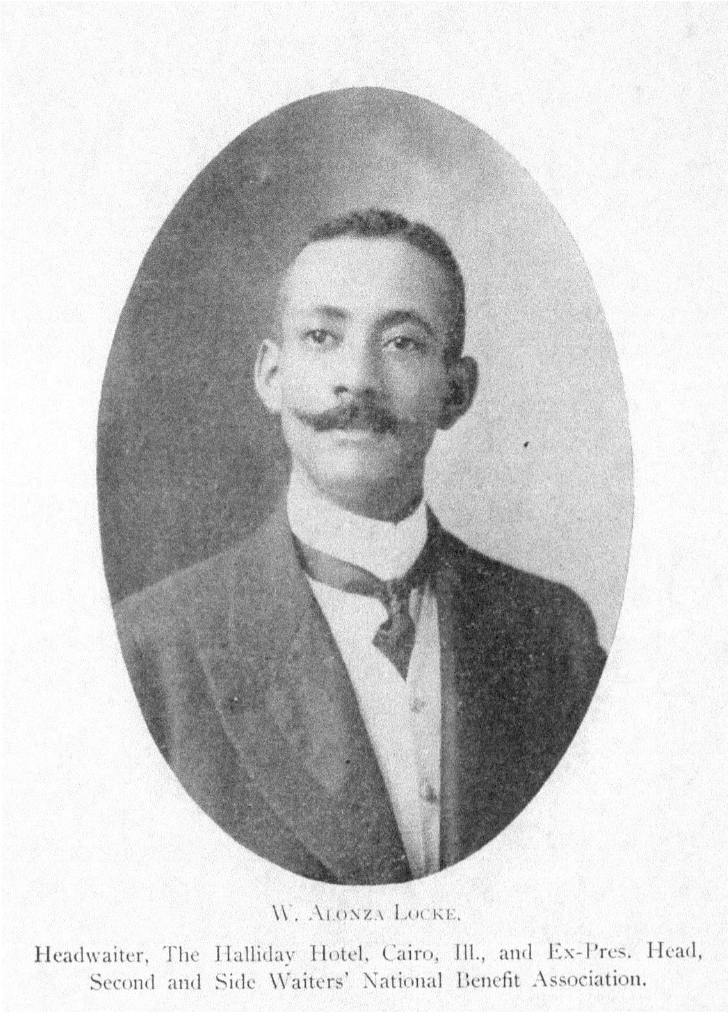

FIGURE 3.3 *W. Alonza Locke. Headwaiter, The Halliday Hotel, Cairo, IL, and Ex-Pres. Head, Second and Side Waiters' National Benefit Association. From E. A. Maccannon,* Commanders of the Dining Room *(New York: Gwendolyn, 1904), 24.*

was an arrangement that had emerged from the tradition of black domestic service in the South.[65] Waiting on tables seemed to constitute a symbolic disempowerment, an "acceptance of racial subordination," as historian Christopher Reed notes. The ritual display of servility, performed in public, was an integral part of the dining experience. "An effective waiter," Reed explains, "conferred on the diner an elevation in social status, even if just for an hour and even if undeserved by social rank."[66]

In a larger context and seen from the perspective of black waiters, things appear in a different light. As Morris's example shows, African American dining room staff focused on much more than on their performances of servility. Black Chicago waiters formed labor organizations in the 1890s. To protest unfair treatment and demand higher wages, they went on strike several times.[67] In the years around 1900, black waiters of elite hotels perceived themselves as part of the new black middle class—a class developing new concepts of African American masculinity.[68] A few decades later, the Brotherhood of Sleeping Car Porters signed the first labor contract ever negotiated with an African American union. Like dining room waiters, sleeping car porters had to perform in an extremely servile mode. And yet, their political success was extremely significant.[69]

Commanders of the Dining Room does not tell the story of a similar breakthrough. It does reflect, however, on the tension between performances of servility and new modes of agency. Maccannon published his collection at a crucial time in African American intellectual history. As one of the leading late nineteenth-century black intellectuals, Booker T. Washington emphasized the necessity of black emancipation in a tone widely perceived as nonconfrontational and accommodating. Challenging Washington's position in the very first years of the twentieth century, W. E. B. DuBois stressed the significance of protest and militancy. In contrast to Washington's preference for invisible, quiet negotiations, he argued for open black protest in the public sphere.[70] DuBois's concept of African American double consciousness helped turn black intellectuals into figures of cultural visibility.[71]

Reflecting on the limitations racism posed for waiters, Maccannon's language seems informed by Washington's public performances. It is flowery and often indirect. But *Commanders of the Dining Room* can also be seen as an example of the new civil rights strategies outlined by DuBois. Maccannon's book explicitly aims to increase visibility for the headwaiters themselves and for the author's critique of the racist system shaping service careers. In this context, the photographs displaying the waiters are more than mere illustrations. They turn into arguments in a larger discourse exploring race and power. A few decades later, Sartre's and Orwell's texts would focus on the French waiter's movements, servile body language, and gestures. In contrast, the photographs in the 1904 volume show waiters at rest and in authoritative poses. The most conspicuous elements of a study conceiving of black servers as "commanders" or "superintendents," they emphasize the central thrust of Maccannon's argument. Discussing photographs of black Civil War soldiers, Maurice O. Wallace argues that these images produced "the first possibility of an imagined national black manhood."[72] While the portraits Maccannon collects do not possess the same kind of cultural relevance, they should be seen as parts of a much larger movement toward African American agency.

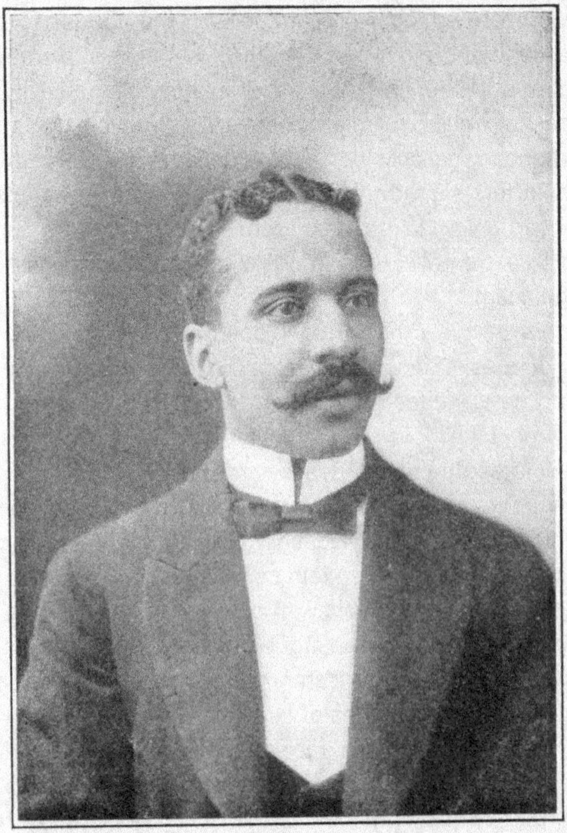

JOHN A. GLOSTER,
Headwaiter, Hotel Sterling, Wilkes Barre, Pa.

FIGURE 3.4 *John A. Gloster, Headwaiter, Hotel Sterling, Wilkes Barre, PA. From E. A. Maccannon,* Commanders of the Dining Room *(New York: Gwendolyn, 1904), 74.*

In contrast to Orwell's and Sartre's observations, this early twentieth-century collection thus indicates how service work and political power are linked in multiple ways. Usually, the waiter appears as a solitary figure. Literary, journalistic, or philosophical texts construct associations around him. In Maccannon's work, writers' associations are much less important than the actual waiters' association initiating the volume: the Head, Second, and Side Waiters' National Benefit Association. The account does not link inauthentic

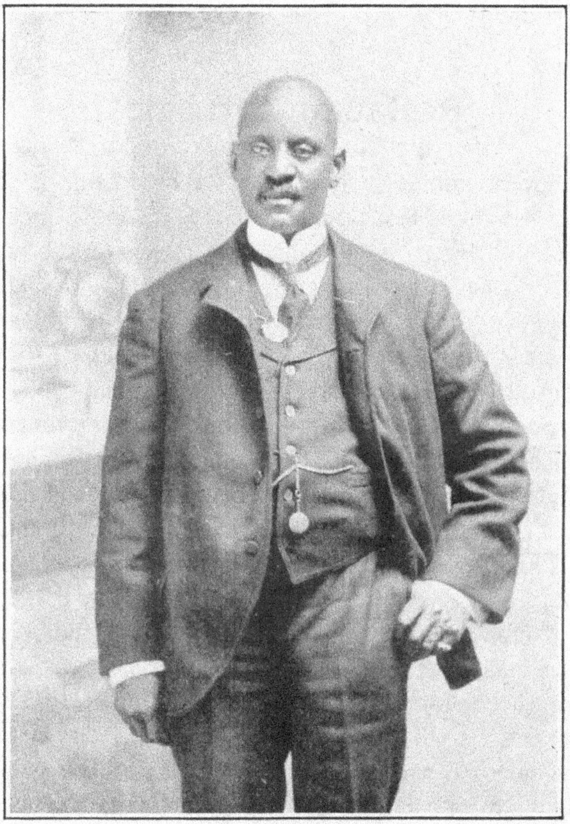

C. M. Farrar.

Treasurer Head, Second and Side Waiters' National Benefit Association.

Headwaiter Merchant Club, Baltimore, Md.

FIGURE 3.5 *C. M. Farrar, Treasurer Head, Second and Side Waiters' National Benefit Association. Headwaiter Merchant Club, Baltimore, MD. From E. A. Maccannon,* Commanders of the Dining Room *(New York: Gwendolyn, 1904), 62.*

service work to automaton identities. Any sort of distinction between performance and authentic personhood is cast aside. *Commanders of the Dining Room* investigates performances only, those of servility and those of authority. It turns into an act of "voluntary inservitude," to echo Michel Foucault's definition of critique.[73] And it could be read as a characteristically African American work—if we follow Kevin Young's distinction between "the white-based construction of authentication" and the "counterfeit or fictional or alternate realities" established in black writing by authors "storying [their] way out of the very bounds of fact and fiction."[74]

Restaurant struggles

After the acknowledgments section, the table of contents, and the preface, the book begins with the first chapter and its first line. This reads, " 'So you take it up the ass?' Benny asks me." What follows for the next half page is homophobic banter and the narrator's triumphant rhetorical comeback ("I don't take it up the butt . . . . But your wife does. Tell her I said hi.").[75] The setting is a restaurant kitchen in a tony New York suburb.

In this mode, *Waiter Rant* begins, a book whose subtitle announces the "confessions of a cynical waiter." And yet, much has been confessed already. Steve Dublanica, a waiter, started to blog about his work experiences in 2004. According to the book jacket, his public diary at www.WaiterRant.net was seen as "the voice for many of the two million waiters in the United States."[76] Published in 2008, Dublanica's memoir transforms the blog into a full-blown narrative of a man beginning to serve tables in his early thirties, working in elite New York-area restaurants, reflecting on service, the culinary world—and on his own masculinity.

Once more, *Waiter Rant* presents the waiter as writer, more than a century after Maccannon's *Commanders of the Dining Room*. The gulf could not be wider. Maccannon and his protagonists emphasize hierarchies and values. They imagine the male server as a figure of power, authority, and immense respectability. Jockeying for attention in early twenty-first-century American culture, Dublanica designs his public persona as rough, rebellious, and cynical. This may be very much at odds with the emotional performances service work requires. But Dublanica notes that he is no stranger to "psychological warfare." It is a kind of warfare that does not aspire to great subtlety. Dublanica calls the dropping of "a silent and deadly fart next to a problematic table" a "nifty chemical weapon" in his power struggles with customers.[77]

While these traits seem adolescent rather than conventionally manly, Dublanica emphasizes the close ties between his prose and American fictions of hard-boiled masculinity. He cites Raymond Chandler as the key influence on his own literary development, praising Chandler's tough "style of wisecracks, metaphors, and sharp lyrical similes."[78] Though the literariness of Dublanica's autobiographical project seems debatable, these references are significant. As Christopher Breu shows, the hard-boiled pose has always served as a "stable site of reader identification" where "rugged individualism" and the "opposition to all forms of collectivity" were performed.[79] Alienated from the mechanism of service work, *Waiter Rant* thus resorts to an accepted shorthand for rebellious manhood. And there are other reasons to call up the hard-boiled style. Competing with successful memoirs by women waiters, Dublanica aims for an exaggerated form of masculinized narrative.[80] Most importantly, his form of dirty restaurant realism imitates one of the most familiar works of the foodie canon, Anthony Bourdain's *Kitchen Confidential*, a chef's memoir evoking kitchen labor as a macho dream space of rebelliousness and intense bodily experience.[81]

In spite of these gestures at radical individualism, Dublanica's narrative does link his life story to collective experiences. The waiter/writer identifies restaurants as "culinary versions of Potemkin villages." He points out that patrons are oblivious to the undocumented migrants preparing the food and clearing the tables. Though in full view, economic injustice will be ignored by the customers. "They don't care," Dublanica states, "that the bus girls might not have enough money for food or that their waiter's sweating the rent." Instead, the author finds that diners, their fantasies shaped by the Food Network, take culinary establishments solely as places catering to their sensual desires. They do not register that "restaurants are places where people struggle to make a living."[82] In these passages, *Waiter Rant* functions like Orwell's 1930s prose. It challenges pretense, however bluntly, in order to establish a critique of the restaurant business. This time, though, the waiter is part of the crowd rather than a player in the performance attacked.

Viewed in a larger early twenty-first-century framework, *Waiter Rant* makes significant points. Employing 10 percent of the American workforce, selling products each year that add up to more than $600 billion, the US restaurant industry still relies on extremely low wages that subsidize the cost of food for the consumer. The average earnings of restaurant workers would force a family to live below the poverty line. The minimum wage for waiters and waitress is significantly lower than the overall minimum wage. This makes servers utterly dependent on tips. Critic and chef Laurie Woolever lists numerous incidents, illegal practices, and structural deficiencies that exacerbate economic injustice and worker disenfranchisement in the restaurant industry.[83] More extensively, Saru Jayaraman's account *Behind the Kitchen Door* explores working conditions and wage theft across the American culinary landscape. Though often assumed to reap the profits of the restaurant world's inequalities, male servers are among the employees in poverty whose plight Jayaraman portrays.[84] Clearly, then, the men Maccannon called "commanders of the dining room" still find themselves in ambivalent positions. They operate in a culinary scene shaped as much by performances of rebellious authenticity as by the pressures exerted on a disempowered emotional proletariat. Though they may not all be as philosophically inclined as Hemingway's hero, their intellectual history seems far richer than Orwell and Sartre suggest.

Notes

Roland Barthes, "Pour une psycho-sociologie de l'alimentation contemporaine," *Annales: Économies, Sociétés, Civilisations* 16, no. 5 (1961): 977–86. Cited here is the English version, "Toward a Psychosociology of Contemporary Food Consumption," in *Food and Culture: A Reader*, ed. Carole Counihan and Penny Van Esterik (1997; New York: Routledge, 2008), 29.

1 Ernest Hemingway, "A Clean, Well-Lighted Place," in *Winner Take Nothing* (New York: Scribner's, 1933), 22.

2 Hemingway, "Clean, Well-Lighted Place," 23. There is a tight connection between the figure of the waiter, in charge of the café as a clean and rigidly organized territory, and the writer, Hemingway, responsible for a similarly well-ordered area: the literary text.

3 See Haley on elite late nineteenth-century restaurants or hotel dining rooms where waiters remained beside one specific table—waiting; Andrew P. Haley, *Turning the Tables: Restaurants and the Rise of the American Middle Class, 1880–1920* (Chapel Hill: University of North Carolina Press, 2011), 35.

4 Joanne Finkelstein, *Fashioning Appetite: Restaurants and the Making of Modern Identity* (London: Tauris, 2014), 69–70.

5 Cameron Lynne Macdonald and Carmen Sirianni, "The Service Society and the Changing Experience of Work," in *Working in the Service Society*, ed. Cameron Lynne Macdonald and Carmen Sirianni (Philadelphia: Temple University Press, 1996), 3.

6 Joanne Finkelstein, "Waiters and Waitresses," in *Encyclopedia of Food and Culture, vol. 3*, ed. Solomon H. Katz (New York: Scribner, 2003), 508; for a more community-oriented reading of restaurants, see: Karla A. Erickson, *The Hungry Cowboy: Service and Community in a Neighborhood Restaurant* (Jackson: University Press of Mississippi, 2009).

7 For a contemporary exception to the rule, see Alain Claude Sulzer's novel *A Perfect Waiter* (New York: Bloomsbury, 2008), a work with obvious intertextual relations to Thomas Mann's novel of the con man (and waiter) Felix Krull. See: Thomas Mann, *Die Bekenntnisse des Hochstaplers Felix Krull* (Frankfurt: Fischer, 1954). For the most important exception to the scholarly disregard for male waiters, consult Gerald Mars and Michael Nicod, *The World of Waiters* (London: Allen & Unwin, 1984).

8 Mitchell Davis, "Restaurant Critics and Food Columnists," in *The Oxford Encyclopedia of Food and Drink in America, vol. 3*, ed. Andrew F. Smith (Oxford: Oxford University Press, 2004), 119. See also: Robert Sietsema, "Everyone Eats . . .: But That Doesn't Make You a Restaurant Critic," *Columbia Journalism Review* (February 2, 2010), accessed May 18, 2016, http://www.cjr.org/feature/everyone_eats.php.

9 See: Tim Stark, *Heirloom: Notes from an Accidental Tomato Farmer* (New York: Broadway, 2008).

10 Frances Donovan, *The Woman Who Waits*, 1920 (New York: Arno, 1974), 140.

11 William Foote Whyte, *Human Relations in the Restaurant Industry* (1948; New York: Arno, 1977), 127.

12 Whyte notes how waitresses "appear to subordinate themselves to customers and at the same time learn to manipulate the people and the situation to their advantage." He calls this a form of "social learning" that enables waitresses "to move up in the world" (Whyte, *Human Relations*, 120).

13 Greta Foff Paules, "Resisting the Symbolism of Service among Waitresses," in *Working in the Service Society*, ed. Cameron Lynne Macdonald and Carmen Sirianni (Philadelphia: Temple University Press, 1996), 287. See also: Paules, *Dishing It Out: Power and Resistance among Waitresses in a New Jersey Restaurant* (Philadelphia: Temple University Press, 1991).

14 Studs Terkel, *Working: People Talk About What They Do All Day and How They Feel About What They Do* (New York: New Press, 1974), 294.

15 Alison Owings, *Hey Waitress! The US from the Other Side of the Tray* (Berkeley: University of California Press, 2004), 4.

16 Leon Elder and Lin Rolens, *The Waitress: America's Unsung Heroine* (Santa Barbara: Capra, 1985); Stephan Schacher, *Plates and Dishes: The Food and Faces of the Roadside Diner* (Princeton: Princeton Architectural Press, 2005); Candacy A. Taylor, *Counter Culture: The American Coffee Shop Waitress* (Ithaca, NY: Cornell University Press, 2009).

17 Owings, *Hey Waitress!* 3.

18 Andrew P. Haley, *Turning the Tables: Restaurants and the Rise of the American Middle Class, 1880–1920* (Chapel Hill: University of North Carolina Press, 2011), 37.

19 Dorothy Sue Cobble, *Dishing It Out: Waitresses and Their Unions in the Twentieth Century* (Urbana: University of Illinois Press, 1992), 21.

20 Haley, *Turning the Tables*, 178.

21 Owings, *Hey Waitress!* 3.

22 Leon Elder, "Foreword," in *The Waitress: America's Unsung Heroine*, 7.

23 See Haley on drilling and the "military style chain of command" that dominated early nineteenth-century service work in restaurants and hotel dining rooms (*Turning the Tables*, 35).

24 Arlie Hochschild, *The Managed Heart: Commercialization of Human Feeling* (Berkeley: University of California Press, 1983), 20.

25 Darren Nixon, "'I Can't Put a Smiley Face On': Working-Class Masculinity, Emotional Labour and Service Work in the 'New Economy'," *Gender, Work, and Organization* 16, no. 3 (2009): 319.

26 Jürgen Martschukat and Olaf Stieglitz, "*'Es ist ein Junge!' Einführung in die Geschichte der Männlichkeiten in der Neuzeit* (Tübingen: Edition Diskord, 2005), 132–5.

27 Ronnie J. Steinberg and Deborah M. Figart, "Emotional Labor since *The Managed Heart*," *Annals of the American Academy of Political and Social Science* 561 (1999): 22.

28 Cameron Lynne Macdonald and David Merrill, "Intersectionality in the Emotional Proletariat: A New Lens on Employment Discrimination in Service Work," in *Service Work: Critical Perspectives*, ed. Marek Korczynski and Cameron Lynne Macdonald (London: Routledge, 2008), 125 and 130.

29 Elaine J. Hall, "Smiling, Deferring, and Flirting: Doing Gender by Giving 'Good Service'," *Work and Occupations* 20 (1993): 452–71.

30 Steinberg and Figart, "Emotional Labor," 9; Claudia Benthien, "Das Maskerade-Konzept in der psychoanalytischen und kulturwissenschaftlichen Theoriebildung," in *Männlichkeit als Maskerade: Kulturelle Inszenierungen vom Mittelalter bis zur Gegenwart*, ed. Claudia Benthien and Inge Stephan (Weimar: Böhlau, 2003), 48.

31 See: Allyson Nadia Field, "Expatriate Lifestyle as Tourist Destination: *The Sun Also Rises* and Experiential Travelogues of the Twenties," *Hemingway Review* 25, no. 2 (2006): 29–43.

32 Mark Pittenger, *Class Unknown: Undercover Investigations of American Work and Poverty from the Progressive Era to the Present* (New York: New York University Press, 2012), 3–4.

33 George Orwell, *Down and Out in Paris and London* (1933; Orlando: Harvest, 1961).

34 George Orwell, *The Road to Wigan Pier* (1937; London: Penguin, 2014), 20; see Patai on effeminate "softness", rather than poverty, as an "abyss" Orwell explores here (Daphne Patai, *The Orwell Mystique: A Study in Male Ideology* [Amherst: University of Massachusetts Press, 1984], 94).

35 Orwell, *Road*, 28–9.

36 Orwell, *Road*, 29.

37 Orwell, *Down*, 68.

38 Orwell, *Down*, 118.

39 Ibid.

40 Desmond MacCarthy, "Foreword," in *Coming, Sir! The Autobiography of a* Waiter (London: Harrap, 1937), 8.

41 Ibid.

42 Orwell, *Road*, 215.

43 Jean-Paul Sartre, *Being and Nothingness: An Essay on Phenomenological Ontology* (1943; London: Methuen, 1969), 59.

44 Sartre, *Being and Nothingness*, 49.

45 Hazel E. Barnes, "Key to Special Terminology," in Sartre, *Being and Nothingness*, 629.

46 Sartre, *Being and Nothingness*, 59; on the ambiguities in this chapter from *Being and Nothingness*, see D. Z. Phillips, "Bad Faith and Sartre's Waiter," *Philosophy* 56, no. 215 (1981): 30. See Appelbaum for an in-depth and restaurant-specific reading of Sartre's thoughts; Robert Appelbaum, *Dishing it Out: In Search of the Restaurant Experience* (London: Reaktion, 2011), 87–92.

47 Sartre, *Being and Nothingness*, 9–10.

48 Sartre, *Being and Nothingness*, 10.

49 Sartre, *Being and Nothingness*, 59–60.

50 Steinberg and Figart, "Emotional Labor," 14–15.

51 George Cotkin, *Existential America* (Baltimore: Johns Hopkins University Press, 2003), 7–8.

52 Grace Hale, *A Nation of Outsiders: How the White Middle Class Fell in Love with Rebellion in Postwar America* (Oxford: Oxford University Press, 2011), 307–8.

53 Alison Pearlman, *Smart Casual: The Transformation of Gourmet Restaurant Style in America* (Chicago: University of Chicago Press, 2013), 8 and 137–8.

54 Josée Johnston and Shyon Baumann, *Foodies: Democracy and Distinction in the Gourmet Foodscape* (New York: Routledge, 2010), 69.

55 Johnston and Baumann, *Foodies*, 181.

56 Dorothy Hamilton, "Preface," in *Chef's Story: 27 Chefs Talk about What Got Them into the Kitchen*, ed. Dorothy Hamilton and Patric Kuh (New York: HarperCollins, 2007), xiv (xii–xv).

57 Pearlman, *Smart Casual*, 85.

58 Pearlman, *Smart Casual*, 86–7.

59 E. A. Maccannon, *Commanders of the Dining Room: Biographic Sketches and Portraits of Successful Head Waiters* (New York: Gwendolyn, 1904), 43–4. Maccannon includes quotations from interviewees like Morris and others.

60 Haley, *Turning the Tables*, 34.

61 Maccannon, *Commanders of the Dining Room*, 2–3.

62 Maccannon, *Commanders of the Dining Room*, 33–4, 35–7, and 45–8.

63 Steven A. Reich, *A Working People: A History of African American Workers since Emancipation* (Lanham, MD: Rowman, 2013), 62. See: Isabel Wilkerson, *The Warmth of Other Suns: The Epic Story of America's Great Migration* (New York: Vintage, 2011).

64 Maccannon, *Commanders of the Dining Room*, 44.

65 Cobble, *Dishing It Out*, 18–20.

66 Christopher R. Reed, *Black Chicago's First Century*, vol. 1, *1833–1900* (Columbia: University of Missouri Press, 2005), 249.

67 Reed, *Black Chicago's First Century*, 251; see also: Margaret Garb, "The Great Chicago Waiters' Strike: Producing Urban Space, Organizing Labor, Challenging Racial Divides in 1890s Chicago," *Journal of Urban History* 40, no. 6 (2014): 1079–98.

68 Martin Summers, *Manliness and Its Discontents: The Black Middle Class and the Transformation of Masculinity, 1900–1930* (Chapel Hill: University of North Carolina Press, 2004); Reed, *Black Chicago's First Century*, 249.

69 Reich, *A Working People*, 95.

70 Cary D. Wintz, "Introduction," *African American Political Thought 1890–1930: Washington, DuBois, Garvey, and Randolph*, ed. Cary D. Wintz

(Armonk: Sharpe, 1996), 5–7. See also DuBois's sociological work on African American "caterers" and their ambivalent relationship to white customers: W. E. B. DuBois, *The Philadelphia Negro: A Social Study*, 1899 (New York: Oxford University Press, 2007), 83–4.

71 Charles Banner-Haley, *From DuBois to Obama: African American Intellectuals in the Public Forum* (Carbondale: Southern Illinois University Press, 2010), 14–15.

72 Maurice O. Wallace, "Framing the Black Soldier: Image, Uplift, and the Duplicity of Pictures," in *Pictures and Progress: Early Photography and the Making of African American Identity*, ed. Maurice O. Wallace and Shawn Michelle Smith (Durham, NC: Duke University Press, 2012), 251.

73 Michel Foucault, "What Is Critique?" in *What Is Enlightenment?*, ed. James Schmidt (Berkeley: University of California Press, 1996), 386.

74 Kevin Young, *The Grey Album: On the Blackness of Blackness* (Minneapolis: Graywolf, 2012), 27–8.

75 Steve Dublanica, *Waiter Rant: Thanks for the Tip—Confessions of a Cynical Waiter* (New York: HarperCollins, 2008), 1–2.

76 Dublanica, *Waiter Rant*, cover jacket.

77 Dublanica, *Waiter Rant*, 182.

78 Dublanica, *Waiter Rant*, 82.

79 Christopher Breu, *Hard-Boiled Masculinities* (Minneapolis: University of Minnesota Press, 2005), 176.

80 See: Debra Ginsberg, *Waiting: The True Confessions of a Waitress* (New York: HarperCollins, 2000); Phoebe Damrosch, *Service Included: Four-Star Secrets of an Eavesdropping Waiter* (New York: HarperCollins, 2007).

81 Anthony Bourdain, *Kitchen Confidential: Adventures in the Culinary Underbelly* (London: Bloomsbury, 2000).

82 Dublanica, *Waiter Rant*, 101.

83 Laurie Woolever, "High-End Food, Low-Wage Labor," *Dissent* (Spring 2012), accessed May 16, 2016, https://www.dissentmagazine.org/article/high-end-food-low-wage-labor.

84 Saru Jayaraman, *Behind the Kitchen Door* (Ithaca, NY: IRL/Cornell University Press, 2013), 85–93.

4

The geography of silence: Food and tragedy in globalizing America

Bryant Simon

Emmett Roe did not care if people whispered about his boxy crew cut or his rumpled jacket. He did not mind if they groused about the ramshackle appearance of his dingy and nearly windowless factory. He just wanted people to stay out of his business, and he did whatever he could to maintain that silence. His drive for anonymity was a kind of metaphor for the larger silence he worked to create.

On the surface, Roe processed chickens, turning chunks of industrially slaughtered meat into nuggets and tenders. But even more, he manufactured silence. Silence, for him and many like him in the relentlessly competitive, labor-intensive nonbranded food industry, was the surest way to garner cheap, tractable labor, and cheap labor was the only way he thought he could stay in business. But Roe knew that he could not produce the silence he needed on his own. He needed the strategic cooperation of government officials at all levels.

To find the cheapest labor and most indifferent government, Roe made in the 1980s what the historian Jefferson Cowie has called a "capital move."[1] In order to keep his business afloat and his authority on the shop floor intact, Roe left one locale where workers had acquired agency through their own organizing efforts and the backing of state regulators, and relocated to another place where labor was cheaper, inexpensive enough that abandoning the fixed costs of an existing factory made rational economic sense. But cheapness came not just in wage rates. It also came through eliminating the "voice" or effective agency of workers.[2] This was not only about shop floor struggles. This was also about place. For Roe, the ideal place was one with a labor surplus that limited workers' options. These were precisely the kinds of places where employers could grab a near monopoly over crucial forms of public agency and keep the regulatory state at arm's length. That combination of control and distance was what silence meant to Roe, that was what he was trying to manufacture in Hamlet, North Carolina, a space to run his factory as cheaply as he could with as few direct challenges and interventions from outside as possible.

Roe's move of his factory from the North of the United States to the South was, then, less about physical location than it was about political economy, the political economy of global capital. In the 1980s, Roe conspired with elected officials in Hamlet to carve out a space to generate profits, a space of carefully crafted silence that allowed him to profit from the risk, danger, and precarity of workers. Even though Roe sold his generic, labelless chicken products to restaurants and schools in the American South and relied on domestic labor and products, the capital moves he made epitomized globalization, for more than the transnational flow of goods, services, equipment, and financing, globalization is about the creation of discrete pockets of vulnerable and muted labor, labor that will be abandoned whenever it speaks too loudly and demands too much. In this system, labor operates in realms of manufactured public silence, silence made (and constantly remade) through a pact between employers in competitive industries and state actors desperate for business to solve their own tax and revenue problems. For working people, the combination of private and state power acted like a muzzle and put their health and safety at risk. Indeed, nothing marks the turn to globalization more than this critical alliance between industry and government to produce cheap goods and perilous silence, yet ironically, this topic has received little attention from scholars of the global economy or students of contemporary foodways.

Roe's plant was located on a quiet side street in the small town of Hamlet. It blew up in 1991, and twenty-five workers were killed there, trapped behind locked doors. This chapter explores Roe's agency in the run-up to the tragedy, the agency of his state allies, and even the agency of flies. Together, the combined agency of these forces conspired to constrain the voices of regulators and workers. The quiet they produced allowed Roe to remain in business and make inexpensive foods sold to underpaid workers. This, then, is the story of cheap food, and the political economy of strategic silences it depends on, a political economy built and rebuilt around the globe over the last five decades to deliver an endless stream of cheap clothes, sneakers, and snacks.

By the time Roe opened the plant on Bridges Street in Hamlet in 1980, the fifty-year-old had been in the food business for more than twenty years. After a stint in the navy, he got into the restaurant business in his hometown of Troy, New York. By the time he reached his twenties, he had moved into the business of supplying food for restaurants, schools, and other institutional outlets. In 1965, the Empire food company of Troy offered Roe a chance to get ahead, but it meant leaving his hometown to run a chicken-processing plant in Moosic, Pennsylvania, a small town a few miles south of Scranton. At first, Roe tried to operate this plant by winning the loyalty of his workforce.

"He worked with us on the floor," recalled Betty Shotwell, an Empire assembly line employee from 1965 to 1983. "He boned and packed [chicken]. He worked with us as if he was another worker." Each September, Roe threw a clambake for his employees at a picnic area by a lake not far from the plant.

In 1970, Roe left Moosic for the chance to run a chain of fried chicken restaurants.[3] Three years later, that operation went bankrupt and Roe was back in Moosic, and eventually he bought the plant and changed the company's name to Imperial Food Products Incorporated. He started out small, with forty employees, but Roe landed contracts to supply chicken nuggets—what one food writer called the hot dog of the 1980s—to grocery stores and food suppliers in the Mid-Atlantic states. Over the next few years, as the taste for nuggets grew, the business expanded and Imperial tripled its workforce to 120 employees.

As Imperial grew, Roe changed his managerial style. There were no more clambakes and no more filling spots on the line or taking a turn deboning chickens. Between when Roe left Moosic to work in the fast food business and when he returned to buy the plant, plant workers had voted in a union. "He did not like unions," Shotwell recalled. "He just changed. He was more strict."[4] What he was not willing to do was give a voice to his workers or to the government.

Beginning in the 1970s, Roe started to look at trade magazines for new locations for his plant. An advertisement caught his eye. Mello-Buttercup, a North Carolina-based ice cream manufacturer, wanted to sell its 33,000-square-foot Hamlet facility.

Louis A. Corning started Mello-Buttercup as the Corning Quality Ice Cream Company in his hometown of Elmira, New York. Corning began his career as a pharmacist. As a side business, he made ice cream. But soon this became his main occupation, and in 1919, a larger firm scooped up his budding company. The deal paid Corning well, but prohibited him from making ice cream again anywhere within 500 miles of Elmira. So Corning, as his grandson recalled, "picked up a map ... and noticed all the railroad connections in Hamlet." Eventually Buttercup, as he called his new company, employed 150 people at the Bridges Street location. When trucks pulled up full of milk and butter, he paid local kids, often African Americans from the nearby projects, to unload the cargo. He hired college students home for the summer to work inside the plant. Perhaps sensing that his branded product depended on good community relations, Corning regularly socialized with the mayor and gave away five-gallon tubs of ice cream for church socials and bake sales. "People around here had a lot of pride in the Buttercup plant," said Barbara Thomas, whose husband worked as the plant manager. "It felt like it was just a real part of Hamlet."[5]

Facing mounting competition from larger ice cream manufacturers, Corning sold the Buttercup plant to the Coastal Diary Company in 1969. For the next nine years, Coastal ran the business under the Mello-Buttercup name, before shutting the plant down and moving to another location.[6] In 1980, Roe paid $137,000 for the boarded-up factory.[7]

Before he signed the papers, Roe surely did some research about the area surrounding the factory. Hamlet, he knew for starters, would bring him closer to his suppliers. After World War II, farmers across the South took to raising chickens, and their wives and children took jobs eviscerating the birds. By the 1970s, sprawling chicken plants dotted the region and cranked out boneless breasts and thigh parts by the millions. In fact, when Roe bought the Buttercup plant, chicken had become the South's largest agricultural product, bigger than tobacco in North Carolina, peanuts in Georgia, cotton in Mississippi, and all crops combined in Alabama.[8] Roe, of course, knew this and knew that a Hamlet plant would allow him to cut his shipping costs. The new location would also provide cheaper power and a warmer climate that demanded less electricity. But the real draws were the combination of cheaper labor and the ability to do business in a state where political leaders were committed to keeping wages down in order to attract new industries.

When Henry Grady and his followers first painted pictures of a New South in the late nineteenth century, they imagined the newly prosperous states of the defeated Confederacy filled with brick factories threaded together by a network of train lines.[9] Bringing industry to Georgia and Alabama involved more than dreams. Investors wanted something that cost less, so boosters promised an abundant supply of inexpensive labor along with cheap natural resources and raw materials. But even more important, they promised freedom, freedom to exploit the environment and freedom from regulations.

Under these conditions, as Jim Cobb, the leading scholar of southern economic modernization, has explained, "industry could be its own boss." Every generation of New South advocates from the 1890s onward renewed Grady's pledge. Come South, they beseeched prospective employers. When the factory owners moved in a little closer, the recruiters whispered, "We will leave you alone and let your run your businesses just the way you want."

In some ways, the men of the New South pioneered the global phenomenon of the "spatial fix," which David Harvey talked about as so central to the neoliberal turn, long before others did. The region's political leaders, like their counterparts a hundred years later in underdeveloped Bangladesh and Vietnam, faced sharply competitive situations. To give their region a leg up, they let business leaders know that they would keep government out of their affairs and give them the freedom they sought to pursue the highest rates of profit possible, including cheaper labor.[10]

When he first starting looking at the Hamlet site, Roe might have been concerned with Democratic governor James B. Hunt and his commitment to making his state safe for industry and a haven for cheap labor. Hearing one of Hunt's stump speeches on the need for early education and racial reconciliation, Roe could have thought for a moment that he heard discordant strains of liberalism, the same kind of pro-safety net, pro-regulatory state he wanted to avoid. But as he listened longer, he would have figured out that the governor was a worthy heir to the region's New South tradition, which was, in essence a tradition of boosterism and benign neglect.[11]

New South leaders, like Hunt, followed the dictum that what is good for business is good for society. In the Southern context, it meant moving away from agriculture and toward more industry, more factories, and more capital investment. To push this transition, political leaders marshaled the power of the state to attract more business. This meant more money for bridges and roads, for schools (sometimes), and for vocational training programs (more often). And it might mean money for travel. New South backers took to the road in search of investment, targeting firms in competitive industries located in states with well-developed regulatory traditions and a tolerance for unions. Anticipating, again, the neoliberal break of the 1970s with the New Deal order, political leaders like Hunt were not antigovernment. Instead, they saw the government not primarily as a protector of citizens or a regulator of the economy but as a cheerleader trying to sell what they had on a competitive open market to eager investors. Once business came, they promised a government ready and willing to do almost anything to safeguard the interests of industry.

First elected governor in 1976, Hunt became "a tireless pursuer of industry and economic growth."[12] Aided by the state's well-funded Industrial Commission, Hunt went from Pennsylvania to Michigan to Ohio trying, in his words, to convince audiences of "the enormous potential for growth and progress that this state has," telling them, "Our location is ideal; we have a perfect climate, our cities are still livable and manageable; our people are honest, thrifty, and hardworking."[13] On these trips, Hunt or one of his professional job hunters would sweeten deals, offering free access roads and sewer lines, and breaks on taxes and salaries. The efforts of Hunt's team paid off. In his first full year in office in 1978, North Carolina added 24,000 industrial jobs. Over the next seven years, the state attracted $41 billion in investment in new factories.[14]

Hunt did not limit himself to the United States on his recruitment trips. In 1978, the governor, several aides, and a television crew headed to Germany on a $30,000 junket in search of new investment. Along the way, they stopped in Ahrensburg to announce that the BeA Fasteners Company—makers of furniture industry clasps—would open a $1.3 million plant in Hamlet. A company spokesperson explained that the firm chose North Carolina because of its "good transportation network and attractive industrial climate."[15] What he did not say was that the state promised to pay half of its plant manager's salary for five years.[16]

Hunt did not mention the insider deal either when he came to Hamlet for a ribbon-cutting ceremony. "I don't have to tell you what it means to Hamlet to have this plant here," the governor maintained. He continued, "Hamlet knows what it's like to have a booming economy, and then lose jobs. This plant is another step forward. [W]hen the second shift is added ... there may be as many as 128 employees. That translates into more tax revenues ... more good paychecks ... and better lives for families." Hamlet, he said, represented other small towns eager for outside investment. "This is what we want for so many of the small towns in North Carolina," the governor asserted, "a chance to grow, yet retain the qualities that make them such good places to live and raise families in."[17]

Roe arrived in Hamlet a couple of years after the BeA plant opened. No one from the Industrial Commission took him out for a dinner and promised to pay the salary of his plant manager.[18] That does not mean Roe did not hear Governor Hunt's probusiness messages or the similar messages of local leaders. Perhaps Roe read the glossy brochure titled "Greetings From Progressive Hamlet." As he flicked through the pages, he might have noticed the section headed "Climate and Farming," and read that "poultry was fast becoming an important fact of life in the area." The brochure's back cover touted Hamlet as "an attractive site for business" with "labor potential," because it was "populated ... with farm people who are native born."[19] Investors like Roe believed that growing up on a farm bred an individualism that inoculated laborers against "collective action." Hamlet officials turned this notion about farm families into a recruitment tool, telling investors that the community was filled with people "who work closely together in their church and Sunday School"—people, Roe read, who kept quiet.[20]

As Roe did his research, he found out what Governor Hunt meant when he said, "Hamlet knows what it's like to have a booming economy, and then lose jobs." The Buttercup factory stood just up the street from the city's Queen Anne-style train depot. Everything in Hamlet was near the station. That is because Hamlet was not that big, only five square miles, and was home to just over 4,500 people in 1980. But more to the point, everything in the town was close to the station because just about every business in the city was there due to the railroad.

Hamlet residents often said there would not have been a Hamlet without the railroad. Founded in 1870, at the intersection of two small rail lines, the town grew over the years into a busy transportation hub. In 1897, the Seaboard Air Railroad moved its headquarters to town. Thirty years later, forty trains rumbled in and out of Hamlet every day.[21] North of the depot, Seaboard built an extensive maintenance shop, followed by a massive roundhouse, then a shipping yard, and finally, a sprawling classification yard. Eventually, seventy-two separate tracks crisscrossed Hamlet. While passenger trains came in the morning and afternoon, most of the trains coming through were freight trains, hauling shirts made in Passaic to Atlanta's department stores and pine planks from South Georgia to High Point's furniture factories.

"My recollection was," wrote Tom Wicker, the award-winning *New York Times* columnist, who was born in Hamlet in 1926, the same year jazz legend John Coltrane was born there, "that practically everyone worked for the railroad."[22] In fact, the railroad employed 3,000 people, a number that added up to almost two-thirds of the town's population. With a virtual monopoly over moving goods across the United States, the railroads piled up hefty profits, turning owners into robber barons and stockholders into stout men in black suits. In this rather uncompetitive industry, managers could easily pass some of the profits on to their workers. And they needed to, because working on the railroad required skill and training. Hoping to gain the loyalty of the workforce, the railroads offered, especially to white men, lifetime employment, steady wages, and unemployment and health benefits. Most important, they tolerated unions and allowed laborers to have a voice in work rules and safety regulations. They also tolerated a role for the state in setting freight rates and passenger schedules.

With its union protections and decent pay, railroad work was the best job a man without a college degree or a family name could get in North Carolina.[23] The money made by engineers and operators spread all over the town. White railroad workers owned roomy houses with manicured lawns and wide front porches. Over time, they moved their families onto curvy streets into what passed for Hamlet's suburbs. The houses owned by these working people had pools in the back and fishing boats parked in the front.

Even Hamlet residents who did not work for the railroads benefited from them. Carpenter J. L. Dooley built and repaired the sturdy homes inhabited by Seaboard engineers and mechanics. W. R. Bosnal and Company manufactured crossties and switches and hired dozens of local men. Before the wide use of refrigerated cars, the Hamlet Ice Company employed fifty men to make blocks of ice and deliver them to the yards to keep Florida fruits and New Jersey vegetables cool and fresh in transit. During World War I, vendors took buckets of fried chicken from McEachern's Hotel, an African American-owned rooming house, down to the station and sold them to hungry black soldiers on troop trains who were not permitted to eat at Main Street's whites-only lunch counters.[24]

Railroad workers' paychecks and what they spent around town contributed to the growth of local businesses and built Hamlet's civic culture of tall churches with stained glass windows and pipe organs. They smoothed out Little League fields and erected center field scoreboards. They built a hospital twice the size of the facility in neighboring and more populous Rockingham that patients from Charlotte and Greensboro traveled to when they fell ill. Laborers and their spouses roamed Main Street, shopping at the stores that lined it during the day and going to the movie houses and restaurants at night.

Beginning in the 1960s, Hamlet's textured economic world of leisure, buying, and worship began to unravel. Work started to disappear. Interstates and highways began to cut across North Carolina. Truckers carried trailers full of cotton bales, mail sacks, live chickens, and loaves of Wonder Bread from the farms to the factories to the cities. At a time when high-end industries and creative-class talent gravitated toward urban centers with universities and interstate highways, Hamlet, "two hours from everywhere," as one local put it, started to die a slow death, one that peripheral places across the global would endure in the postwar era and one that left them susceptible to the promises of anyone offering a few jobs and a little bit of investment.[25]

The signs of decline were all over Hamlet as the railroad left and the town's economy effectively shifted from a developed one to an underdeveloped one. By the 1980s, despite Hamlet Hospital's presence, Richmond County had less than half as many physicians per capita as the rest of the state. Teenage pregnancy and infant mortality were on the rise. Between 1970 and 1980, the proportion of older residents and high school dropouts climbed in Hamlet as the town's best and brightest and most educated went away to school and did not come back except to visit over the summer or at Christmas.[26]

Starting in the early 1970s, Hamlet and scores of other small towns across the country started to unwind, to borrow journalist George Packer's phrase about the state of America in recent years. As they did, these places began to mimic Food Lion and Walmart. Working people, like these stores, survived on the cheap. Prices were lower, but so were wages. With the railroad laying off hundreds of men, there were fewer well-paying jobs in town, and more part-time work and full-time jobs that paid part-time wages. As pay envelopes shrunk, working people demanded lower prices. As they did, Main Street, with its local shops, became too expensive, a retail anachronism of an older time. But the death of the downtown and the rise of box stores played, at the same time, into the hands of Roe and his relentless focus on silence and on the bottom line. It provided him, at once, with hungry customers in search of cheap calorie-rich foods, like the fatty nuggets and tenders he produced at his plant, and a pool of desperate laborers in need of a job, any job.[27]

It was not just the railroads that were in decline. Nearby Rockingham had been a textile center since the Civil War. By the end of World War II, ten mills, employing more than ten-thousand people, churned out shirts and underwear for Hanes, Fruit of the Loom, and Burlington Industries. Forty years later, boxer shorts from Mexico and T-shirts from Guatemala filled the racks at the K-Mart store on the highway. Local jobs tending looms and spindles went South too. When Roe bought the Buttercup plant, only a few local textile factories were still open, and by that point, several of them had been so thoroughly automated that they did not need but a few hundred semiskilled workers to keep the line moving.[28]

As work went overseas and tractor-trailers replaced railroad locomotives hauling goods, jobs that allowed men to play the part of the breadwinner, supporting a family and paying a mortgage, were harder to find in Hamlet. Statistics told part of the story of the area's industrial decline. When Roe bought the ice cream plant in 1980, unemployment in North Carolina stood at 6.5 percent.[29] In Hamlet and Rockingham, it was 9.4 percent. By 1982, it had climbed to 14.7 percent, making just about any job in the area, even if it was a hot and filthy one that left your back and wrists throbbing, tolerable, if not desirable. "Round Hamlet, things are slow and people are poor and they are thankful for any job they can get," observed Alphonce Anderson, whose wife, Peggy, died in the Imperial Food Products fire.[30]

Joblessness, Roe surely knew, meant increased competition for work at his plant, lower labor costs, and less room for open dissent. Plus it meant, he would not need to build loyalty or listen to his laborers. Hamlet was now a place with an abundance of workers, most without a lot of options. As the railroad scaled back, union men had to work for less. At the same time, they had to compete with out-of-work textile workers for area positions.[31] In a pattern repeated across the United States in the 1970s, as men made less, families mobilized more of their resources. Women entered the paid labor force in Hamlet, just like everywhere else, in growing numbers. In 1970, 30 percent of women in the United States with children under six years old held paying jobs. By 1985, more than half did.[32] More overall workers in the labor pool—a by-product of the collapse of the nation's primary industries like railroads and steel—drove down wage rates for the least skilled workers, especially as regions and states started to compete with each other for industries.

Roe knew that the drop in railroad jobs put downward pressure on wages. He knew, probably by heart, the county's unemployment statistics, and if he did not, he knew by driving down Main Street that the town's better days were behind it. Hamlet's mayor remembered being excited to have Imperial in town "because of the jobs." Played right, Roe understood, enthusiasm mixed with decay would let him manufacture the silence he wanted. He knew that this quiet would come cheap in a place like Hamlet that was battered by job losses, far from the urban core, and forced into competition with other hard-pressed places for low-paying industries. This also meant that state and local officials, themselves in search of revenues, would assist him in keeping unions at bay and workers quiet.

"We should maintain our good business climate," Hunt declared in 1980, adding, "I strongly support the right-to-work law."[33] He never condemned unions outright, but he did not support them either. He appointed officials to oversee business recruitment to the state with similar views. "North Carolinians are as bright as anyone else," Larry D. Cohick, Hunt's economic development chief told a reporter, adding, "I would guess that if they as a group wanted unions, the state would have them. If union leaders could demonstrate the need for unions, you would have them."[34]

By 1990, North Carolina emerged as a leader in the pitched national battle, often between states, for revenues and jobs. Quite remarkably, the one-time agricultural powerhouse had become the most industrialized state in the country. That meant it had more factory jobs per capita than Michigan, Ohio, or Pennsylvania. Perhaps not surprisingly given emerging economic trends, it also had the nation's stingiest worker compensation system, lowest average hourly wage rate, and lowest percent of unionized laborers.[35]

By this time, Richmond County, where Hamlet was located, was no more welcoming to unions than the rest of the state. Neil Cadieu edited the local paper and worked in industrial recruitment. When employers looking to relocate their factories asked him about unions, he assured them "in emphatic terms" that if they moved to the country they would not have to deal with organized labor.[36]

No doubt, Roe relished the silence that Cadieu and Hamlet promised, but he never let his guard down. He worked hard to maintain his anonymity to the point that he shunned local elites. He did not glad hand with city leaders or sponsor a youth sports team or give away boxes of chicken tenders for church socials. The Imperial plant never even had a sign over its door. "It was a half mile from downtown," a labor safety advocate remembered, "and you just got the sense that it was something that someone wanted to keep out of sight."[37] No balloons or ribbon-cutting ceremonies accompanied Imperial's opening. Roe's arrival in town did not even make the local newspaper. When representatives from the Richmond County United Way asked permission to solicit contributions from Imperial workers, Roe said no. He did not want any prying eyes in his plant. Other local leaders got the same chilly reception. The executive director of the Richmond County Chamber of Commerce visited Roe one day to ask if he would join the organization, only to be rebuffed. "It was like I was trying to get him to join the union," he recalled with surprise.[38] Roe did not want anyone to know what he was doing with his business.

Production started slowly at the Imperial plant. It took time to turn the ice cream factory into a food-processing facility. Walls were moved. Additions were built. Coolers and fryers were brought in. Architects did not seem to be involved in any of the renovations. Neither were local officials. Roe never applied for a single building permit, as the law mandated, and no one in Hamlet asked him to comply, even as they surely heard the sound of walls crashing and delivery trucks hauling heavy equipment up the hill to the plant.

After a small fire at the factory in 1983, Roe assured Hamlet officials that he would install a new sprinkler system. No one followed up, but the neglect, again, clued Roe into how things would operate. In need of employers and tax revenues in the absence of the railroad and mills, local leaders would leave him alone and he turned that to his advantage. Processing chicken required prodigious amounts of water and produced a tremendous amount of discarded liquids, yet no one at the outset asked Roe if he had any waste treatment plans. It turned out, it seemed, that Roe did have a plan, a secret plan. He appears to have dug a series of illegal wells inside of his plant that allowed him to take water from the ground and have it processed into waste without charge. But again, no one knocked on Roe's door to find out what was going on, so no one knew about his thievery or wanted to know how he was processing so much chicken without using much water.

It was like a "ghost operation," Ron Niland, the former city manager said. "As long as there weren't any problems and no one was getting hurt, no one paid any attention."[39] This was exactly the sort of "benign neglect," to use Niland's term, Roe wanted. This was why he made the capital move to Hamlet. He wanted to make silence there.

Back in Moosic, though, Roe was not getting the silence he wanted. Fire, again, blew his cover. In 1985, an employee suffered third-degree burns after getting sprayed by hot cooking oil. A local television station featured the story on the nightly news. That is how the Occupational Safety and Health Administration (OSHA) found out about the plant. When an inspector knocked on the Roe's door, he would not let him in. Three months later, the inspector returned with a search warrant. After a careful examination of the plant, he discovered several minor safety violations.

Two years later, another Imperial employee contacted OSHA, complaining of unsafe working conditions. In his February 1987 report on his visit to the plant, Inspector E. F. Donnelly wrote that Roe displayed "utter contempt for OSHA." After combing through the factory, he found six violations, three of them "serious." (Serious was OSHA's term for issues that were noteworthy but not deemed immediately life threatening.)[40] Six months after Donnelly filed his report, OSHA was back at Imperial for a more thorough inspection. Investigators spent ninety-seven hours examining injury logs, checking on safety procedures, observing the way the assembly line and cooker operated, testing fire alarms, and opening and closing safety doors. When they finished, they uncovered thirty-three health and safety violations, fifteen of them serious, including unlit exit signs, blocked exits, and electrical cords lying in pools of water. One employee told the inspector that the plant was "an accident waiting to happen." Despite the severity of the infractions, Imperial was fined only $2,560.[41]

Roe, though, had had enough, enough of OSHA and the state prying into his business, trying to gain a voice in how he ran things. In another hallmark of the silencing that goes with globalization, he moved. He shut down the Pennsylvania plant and moved his entire operation South. His strategy for making money in the new locale: keep government out and labor quiet.

North Carolina law required all new employers of ten or more people to register with OSHA. The agency then put each company into a kind of lottery system. When their number came up, they would get a surprise inspection. (Otherwise, a complaint, like it did in Moosic, would trigger an inspection.) The chances of getting inspected were not high, but you never knew when the regulators might knock on the door, and this in theory encouraged employers to keep their factories safe, clean, and to listen to their employees about working conditions—except for Roe. He never registered with OSHA and avoided the possibility of oversight through another layer of deliberately made silence.[42]

Hamlet officials continued to leave Roe alone. Like so much else about Imperial, the owner's calculated silence only became clear after the deadly fire. Not long after the blaze, Hamlet's tax collector went through the files in her office and found that the city had no listing for personal property or inventory taxes from Imperial, as the law required the company to submit. But no one in city government hassled the company. City leaders did not want to scare them off and see them move to another town.[43] The state

Insurance Department reported, again after the fire, that Imperial never obtained a building permit for the additions it added or the changes it made to the building. Each was a violation of the law, but the laws were not enforced.

Again and again, Roe figured out that no one in the state capitol or the county or the city would make him follow the letter of the law. He was Hamlet's largest private employer, and this was a town, as Governor Hunt admitted on his visit to mark the BeA factory opening, starved for jobs. Practicing the "benign neglect" that town manager Niland talked about, the mayor never even stepped foot in the factory, until after the fire. This indifference continued as Roe ratcheted up production, adding a second shift and hiring more people. Still, no one came to the factory, not even after another small fire broke out there in 1987 and required the fire company to put it out. No one came after the city manager and others finally figured out that Imperial was dumping discarded chicken parts and fat into the city's water supply. At one point, the city had to shut off its water for hours to clean things up. Yet Roe continued to flood the system with waste. Just days before the fire, the city threatened to close down Imperial. Roe stonewalled, and then finally agreed to make a small change to keep local officials out of the plant and from finding out about his system of illegal wells.[44]

The government agency with the most contact with Roe was the United States Department of Agriculture (USDA). On most days, a USDA inspector showed up at Imperial. His job, in a sense, was to speak for consumers and make sure their voices and concerns were heard. He walked past the giant fryer, stuck his head in the freezer, checked the floors for mouse and rat droppings, and peeked around the trash bins for insects. He made sure that workers scrubbed and disinfected the machines and kept rancid meat out of the tenders and nuggets. He noted when workers touched food without washing their hands or grabbed chicken that fell to the floor and put it back on the conveyor belt, as some said Roe, who was always trying to trim costs, ordered them to do.

Two years before the fatal fire, Roe received a stream of notices from the USDA about flies in the plant. He tried to silence them, and government actors, by putting up flytraps and sending workers around with fly swatters. But he could not contain the insects. Flies kept coming in from one of the back doors near the trash dumpster. In July 1991, USDA inspectors complained again to Roe about the fly problem. They noted that workers kept leaving the door near the trash open and flies kept coming in. Frustrated with the company's performance, the USDA threatened to close Imperial down, something Roe couldn't afford.

An Imperial manager outlined the company's final solution to the fly problem. "Outside door to this area," he explained about the part of the plant near the dumpster, "will be locked at all times unless for an emergency."

The USDA inspectors signed off on the scheme and seemed satisfied that Imperial had finally handled its fly problem.[45]

An exit door bolted shut from the outside, however, violated every basic workplace safety rule put on the books in the United States since the fatal Triangle Shirtwaist Factory fire in New York in 1911. "Are you kidding me?" a Cornell University industrial safety expert said after reading the USDA's report.[46] But at the time, the meat inspectors said nothing. The Roes silenced them with a locked exit. Still focused on the meat and the shoppers further down the food chain, the USDA came in and out of the factory most every day between July and September of 1991, knowing that an exit door was locked, keeping the flies out and the workers in.

For Roe, the locked door had an added advantage. Not only would it hinder the flies from coming into the plant and get the USDA out of his business but it would also stop the stealing of boxes of tenders, something that Roe saw as a problem after he caught an employee with $245 worth of fried chicken products in his car in March 1991. After the tenders were discovered, workers detected heightened security at the back door leading to the parking lot. While they said nothing about it publicly, they were again silenced, as theft, as numerous scholars have pointed out, was itself a form of resistance, a way to register discontent and a means of gaining a voice.[47]

In the days and weeks after the fire, the press revealed the USDA's silence about the locked exit door. When asked by reporters why inspectors said nothing about the doors, the USDA's deputy administrator for inspections explained, "We're strictly in there as food safety inspectors."[48]

Meanwhile, OSHA, the agency in charge workplace safety, never visited Roe's North Carolina plant or found the locked doors. Neither did the local fire department. Despite previous fires and talk around town about the dangers inside the plant, local fire officials never inspected Imperial, not even after state law said they had to do so. During its 1991 legislative session, the North Carolina General Assembly passed a measure compelling all of the state's municipal and county governing units to appoint a fire inspector by July 1 of that year. The inspectors were required to apply a new uniform and comprehensive fire code, also effective July 1, in making inspections. But the state did not fund the program. By the summer deadline, only 257 of the state's 613 governmental units had named a fire inspector. Hamlet was one of those places that had not designated anyone for the job. The city and its fire department insisted that they did not have the money to pay for inspections, so they never combed through the city's commercial buildings and factories. As a result, no one ever walked through the Imperial plant slowly enough to notice the bolted door in the back. No one except for the USDA men saw that the Bridges Street factory lacked working sprinklers or well-lit exit signs or that dangerous fluids leaked from connections perilously close to flames not fully covered.[49]

Roe did not just take the silence that local, state, and federal officials gave him, itself a hallmark of globalization and the intentional chipping away at regulation that has accompanied it. He also reinforced silence through how he recruited labor. "I didn't know anybody who worked there," Hamlet's Ruth Land, the wife of a local car dealer, said in 1991. She added, "Just people you didn't know worked down there." Those were exactly the people Roe hired to work for him, people without a voice in the halls of city government. People no one cared about. People without social capital. People easily replaced. Over the years, Roe let officials at the Hamlet unemployment office know when he needed workers. They sent him high school dropouts and people who lived in the public housing project just down the street from the plant. They sent him single women with young children, especially African American women. Over time, Roe cast a wider net. He employed more single mothers from trailer parks and rural enclaves even more depleted than Hamlet who were willing to drive twenty minutes for a minimum-wage job. These, too, were people Land could not see or hear.[50]

"You couldn't complain, you couldn't say anything," an Imperial line worker remarked. If you did, "you were out of there." The lack of employment options and the absence of union representation reinforced workers' silence. Maggie Brown said that although she and her coworkers talked about the wet floors, locked doors, and unmarked exits, she knew of no one who complained to Roe or the plant supervisors. "The managers didn't talk to anyone like they was human," Mary Pouncey said about Imperial. "When you got three or four children, and that is all you have, you can put aside what he says." So she stayed quiet about the plant's unsafe conditions. "They never had a drill ... while I was working there," Pouncey told filmmakers in 1992, "There was no sprinkler system. There was a lot that you knew that wasn't right, but if you complained about it, you got fired."[51]

Line workers sometimes implemented the silence themselves. Ada Blanchard grew up near Hamlet, but during her teens, she ran off to Philadelphia. A failed marriage brought her back to North Carolina in the 1980s. Still, she said she learned up North to speak up for herself. She even referred to herself as a "loudmouth." She talked to her Imperial coworkers about the lack of fire drills and about flash fires that broke out near the gigantic fryer. She wanted to talk to the bosses, but her coworkers stopped her. Every time she was about to say something, they reminded her of the realities of the local political economy. They told her what she already knew, that there were not any other jobs in the area that paid above minimum wage. They told her what the managers told them. If they complained too much, the company would move. Then there would be nothing. Working and keeping a job in small town North Carolina was a lot like keeping a job anywhere in the global South. It meant keeping your mouth shut and keeping the plant's secrets and safety violations locked inside.

Roe was never going to be the first to talk. Even after the deadly fire at his plant in 1991, he remained silent. When a reporter asked him about the locked doors, he shrugged and said he did not know anything. When newsmen tried to slip into Imperial's office across the road from the charred plant, Roe slammed the door in their faces. Asked to confirm that he was, in fact, Emmett Roe, he shot back, "Never mind who I am. It's not important." The reporters persisted. Roe still did not answer, at least not with words. He flashed the middle finger. Roe never spoke with city officials. He never sent the families of the dead or injured a sympathy card. Even as "Wanted for Murder" posters with his picture popped up in union halls and churches around the country, he still said nothing.

At a hearing in his criminal trial on charges of twenty-five counts of involuntary manslaughter, others spoke for Roe. His attorney cut a deal that sentenced him to prison for nearly nineteen years but allowed his son Brad and his son-in-law, James Hair, both of whom worked in Hamlet as supervisors and managers, to walk away free of any charges.[52] When Roe entered the penitentiary in 1995, he said nothing. When he was paroled four and half years later, he said nothing. When he moved into the basement of his son's house outside of Atlanta, he said nothing.

But the silences Roe so carefully created and assiduously maintained in Hamlet were not, unfortunately, out of the ordinary, not then and not now. There is a similar silence that sustains and fuels the global economy, an economy that delivers inexpensive goods and cheap foodstuffs by deliberately and systematically muffling the voices of workers and state regulators so that it can cover up and externalize the true costs of the system. These silences are too often revealed only in moments of tragedy, when workers die in collapsed factories in Bangladesh, burned chicken plants in China, and crumbling and uninspected buildings in Philadelphia.

Notes

1 Jefferson Cowie, *Capital Moves: RCA's Seventy-Year Quest for Cheap Labor* (New York: The New Press, 2001).

2 My thinking here and throughout this essay has been shaped by Albert O. Hirschman's seminal work on agency, *Exit, Voice, and Loyalty: Responses to Decline in Firms, Organizations, and States* (Cambridge, MA: Harvard University Press, 1970).

3 "Hamlet Fire Latest in a Long List of Imperial Setbacks," *Richmond County Daily Journal*, (herein RCDJ), September 16, 1991.

4 C. E. Yandle and Jim Barnett, "The Road to Ruin," *Raleigh News and Observer*, December 10, 1991.

5 Jane Ruffin, "Dreams of Better Days," *Raleigh News and Observer*, December, 9, 1991.

6 Ibid.

7 Yandle and Barnett, "The Road to Ruin."

8 Tony Horwitz, "Nine to Nowhere," *Wall Street Journal*, December 1, 1994; Doug Stark, "The South's Poultry Plants Thrive," *Baltimore Sun*, September 8, 1991; and Hope Shand, "Billions of Chickens: The Business of the South," *Southern Exposure* (November/December 1983), 76–82. On the emergence and timing of the Southern chicken industry, see Kathleen C. Schwartzman, *The Chicken Trail: Following Workers, Migrants, and Corporations Across the Americas* (Ithaca: ILR Press, 2013).

9 Paul Gaston, *The New South Creed: A Study of Southern Myth Making* (Baton Rouge: Louisiana State University Press, 1976).

10 For more on idea of the South as a forerunner of globalization, really, neoliberalism, see James C. Cobb, *The Selling of the South: The Southern Crusade for Industrial Development, 1936–1990* (Urbana: University of Illinois Press, 1993), 229–30; Mary E. Frederickson, *Looking South: Race, Gender, and the Transformation of Labor from Reconstruction to Globalization* (Gainesville: University of Florida Press, 2011) and Leon Fink, *The Maya of Morganton: Work and Community in the Nuevo New South* (Chapel Hill: University of North Carolina Press, 2003). David Harvey, obviously one of the most important scholars of neoliberalism, has written on the Hamlet fire. See his essay "Class Relations, Social Justice, and the Political Geography of Difference," in Harvey, *Justice, Nature and the Geography of Difference* (Cambridge, MA: Blackwell Publishing 1996), 335–56.

11 On Hunt, see Rob Christensen, *The Paradox of Tar Heel Politics: The Personalities, Elections, and Events That Shaped Modern North Carolina* (Chapel Hill: University of North Carolina Press, 2008), 140–50; Paul Luebke, *Tar Heel Politics: Myths and Realities* (Chapel Hill: University of North Carolina Press, 1990), 74–6; Gary Pearce, *Jim Hunt: A Biography* (Winston Salem: James F. Blair Publishers, 2010); and George Tindall, *The Emergence of the New South, 1913–1945* (Baton Rouge: Louisiana State University Press, 1967).

12 Tom Wicker, "A Governor's Dilemma," *New York Times*, December 8, 1991.

13 Address to North Carolina Citizens Association, Raleigh, March 24, 1977, Memory F. Mitchell, ed., *Address and Public Papers of James Baxter Hunt Jr.*, vol. 1, *1977–1981*, (Raleigh: Division of Archives and History, 1982), 83–3. On the larger antiunionism of the region, see Bruce J. Schulman, *The Seventies: The Great Shift in American Culture, Society, and Politics* (New York: Free Press, 2001), 111.

14 Edward Martin, "The Great Divide," *Business North Carolina* (February 2001), 18.

15 News Release from the Governor's Office, "Hunt Announces German Plant to Locate in Richmond County," April 5, 1978, Box 148, Folder, B, Industrial Development, Division of Industrial Commission, James B. Hunt Papers,

NC State Archives, Raleigh; and Memory F. Mitchell, ed., *Addresses and Public Papers of James Baxter Hunt Jr.*, vol. 1, *1977–1981* (Raleigh: Division of Archives and History, 1982), 820. Janet Guyon, "Hamlet to Get German Plant," *Raleigh News and Observer*, April 6, 1978.

16 Lester Suss (President of BeA Fasteners) to Hunt, November 13, 1978, Box 174, Folder, B, Industrial Development, Division of Industrial Commission, James B. Hunt Papers, North Carolina State Archives, Raleigh.

17 Box 279, Folder, Remarks, Ribbon Cutting—BeA Fasteners Company, September 22, 1978, James B. Hunt Papers, North Carolina State Archives, Raleigh.

18 Governor Martin Papers, Governor's Press Office, Press Conference Transcript, 1985–1991, Box 7 Folder—Press Conference Transcript, 9/19/91, North Carolina State Archives, Raleigh. John Hechinger and John Drescher, "Does N.C. Send the Wrong Message," *Charlotte Observer*, October 7, 1991.

19 "Greetings from Progressive Hamlet at the Crossroads of the Carolinas," pamphlet from the Hamlet Depot Museum, Hamlet.

20 James C. Cobb, *The Selling of the South: The Southern Crusade for Industrial Development, 1936–1990* (Urbana and Chicago: University of Illinois Press, 1993), 108.

21 Martha Quillin, "Grief Runs Deep," *Raleigh News and Observer*, September 2, 2001.

22 Gordon Edes, "From Hamlet to Megalopolis: Dodgers' Franklin Seems to Have Arrived to Stay," *Los Angeles Times*, June 18, 1986.

23 On middle-class life and economic security, see Hedrick Smith, *Who Stole the American Dream* (New York: Random House, 2012).

24 Tom Lawton, "The Life and Times of a Railroad Town," *Fayetteville Observer*, February 28, 1982.

25 MDC, Inc. (Chapel Hill, NC), "Three Faces of Rural North Carolina: A Summary Report to the North Carolina Commission on Jobs and Economic Growth" (December 1986), 1, North Carolina Collection, Chapel Hill.

26 MDC Report, "Three Faces," 12. See also Peter A. Coclanis and Louis M. Kyriakoudes, "Selling Which South?: Economic Change in Rural and Small-Town North Carolina in an Era of Globalization, 1940–2007," *Southern Cultures* (Winter 2007), 96; and Jane Ruffin, "A World Apart," *Business North Carolina* (April 1992), 48. See also Patrick J. Carr and Maria J. Kefalas, *Hollowing Out the Middle: The Rural Brian Drain and What It Means for America* (Boston: Beacon Press, 2010).

27 George Packer, *The Unwinding: An Inner History of the New America* (New York: Farrar, Straus, and Giroux, 2013), 105. See also Nelson Lichtenstein, *The Retail Revolution: How Wal-Mart Created a Brave New World of Business* (New York: Metropolitan Books, 2009), 206 and 209.

28 *Mixed Blessings: Richmond County, 1900–2000* (Ellerbe, NC: Richmond County Historical Society, 2000), 123–34; MDC Report, "Three Faces,"

Appendix C, p. 13; and Riley Watson, interviewed by Abbie Covington, August 19, 2009, Hamlet Depot Museum Oral History Project.

29 Ruffin, "A World Apart."

30 Jennifer French Parker, "Poultry Industry's Boom in N.C. Has A Price Tag," *Charlotte Observer*, September 9, 1991.

31 Martha Quillin, "Grief Runs Deep," *Raleigh News and Observer*, September 2, 2001.

32 Schulman, *The Seventies*, 161–2.

33 "The Candidates: Governor, James B. Hunt, Jr," *We the People of North Carolina*, April 1980, 34. See also Hunt to E. G. Matheson, Plant manager, Rheem Manufacturing Company, (Apex), August 23, 1977, Box 38, Folder, Labor Department of, K-Z, James B. Hunt Papers, NC State Archives, Raleigh.

34 "Interview with Larry D. Cohick, The State's New Economic Development Chief," *We the People of North Carolina*, November 1978, 42.

35 "North Carolina Highly Attractive for Manufacturers, National Study Shows," *Chapel Hill News*, February 14, 1982; *A Study of Manufacturing Business Climates of the Forty-Eight Contiguous States of America, 1980* (Chicago: Alexander Grant and Company, 1981).

36 Interview with Neil Cadieu by Abbie Covington, n. d., Hamlet Depot Museum Oral History Project, Hamlet.

37 Letter from Mark Schultz to author, December 18, 2013.

38 Yandle and Barnett, "The Road to Ruin."

39 Letter from Niland to author, May 22, 2014.

40 Yandle and Barnett, "The Road to Ruin."

41 As part of an Freedom of Information Act request, Mark Stelmark to Bryant Simon, October 12, 2012 (in author's possession).

42 "Imperial Never Licensed Operate in N.C.," RCDJ, October 3, 1991.

43 "Hamlet Fire Latest in a Long List of Imperial Setbacks," RCDJ, September 16, 1991. See also City of Hamlet, "The Following Businesses are Listed According to the Amount of Their 1991 Taxes," Hamlet City Hall Records.

44 Letter from Niland to author, May 22, 2014. (See also the water question, City Hall records made available to the author by Abbie Covington, Uncategorized, Hamlet, NC.)

45 These are from the USDA's inspection reports. I obtained these from Steve Riley, a reporter from the *News and Observer*, and they are in the author's possession.

46 Letter from Nellie Brown to author, August 30, 2011.

47 John Drescher and Ken Garfield, "Worker: Doors Kept Locked," *Charlotte Observer*, September 5, 1991. On the politics of theft, see James Scott, *Weapons of the Weak: Everyday Forms of Peasant Resistance* (New Haven, CT: Yale University Press, 1985).

48 Dateline, NBC, n. d., in Charles Becton Files, Personal Collection, Durham; Steve Riley, "US Agency Knew about Locked Door," *News and Observer*,

November 13, 1991; John Hood, "Over-reaction to Hamlet Tragedy Will Only Create Additional Victims," *Atlanta Journal Constitution*, September 3, 1992.

49 Randy Diamond, "Panel Will Consider Fire Inspection Rules," *Raleigh News and Observer*, September 9, 1991.

50 Ruffin, "Dreams of Better Days." On Roe's reliance on "employment services," see the film "Out of the Ashes" (North Carolina Occupational Safety and Health Project, 1994).

51 Paul Taylor, "Ashes and Accusations," *Washington Post*, September 5, 1991; and "Out of the Ashes."

52 "Meat-Plant Owner Pleads Guilty In a Blaze that Killed 25 People," *New York Times*, September 15, 1992; "Owner Gets 20 Years in Fatal Poultry Plant Fire," *Chicago Tribune*, September 15, 1992.

PART THREE

Health

Conditioning originates with the body but goes beyond it. It produces energy . . .; alertness . . ., and relaxation.

ROLAND BARTHES, 1961

5

Making food matter: "Scientific eating" and the struggle for healthy selves

Nina Mackert

"I am feeling very disagreeable but am bound to pull through," Roscoe Maxwell Rhoads wrote in his diary on a late-December day in 1898, at the beginning of what would be a three-and-a-half-month stay at the famous sanitarium in Battle Creek, Michigan.[1] Rhoads was the son of a wealthy, white family from Indiana. At the time, he was eighteen years old and probably neurasthenic.[2] Determined to get well, he was visiting the sanitarium for a second time. The fact that Rhoads chose Battle Creek is significant for two reasons: first, John Harvey Kellogg's sanitarium was *the* place for white elites to find treatment for whatever ailed them.[3] Second, Rhoads was committed to "hygienic eating," a dietary regimen closely associated with the sanitarium. Rhoads was convinced that a proper diet was central to his recovery, and he wrote about this extensively in his diary. His daily entries in the years 1897–1902 and 1916–1918 bear witness to his struggles for health and his attempts to eat right as well as the increasing significance of nutrition and diet in the understanding and practices of health and the self in the decades around 1900.[4]

The years surrounding the turn of the century are considered a crucial time in the history of bodies. An increasing focus on hygiene, physical fitness, and health provided the modern Western ideal of self-conscious and self-controlled individuals with a distinct physique.[5] The question of successful selves became a corporeal one, and it is no coincidence that at the very same time, these selves seemed to be endangered by sickness, racial decline, and the excessive demands of a society in disarray.[6] In recent years, scholars have increasingly turned to the era's nutritional advice, particularly food reform movements, and have highlighted their role in shaping people's understanding of the impact of food on health, body shape, and individual and collective progress.[7] However, historians have rarely looked at the practices of historical actors themselves and how they made sense of food and diet in their daily lives.[8] Rhoads's intense preoccupation with diet and nutrition offers a glimpse into the way new nutritional knowledge shaped people's lives in the Progressive Era.

Born in 1880 in Anderson, Indiana, the fifth child of Abe and Adaline Rhoads, Maxwell grew up in an upper-class white family and had enough leisure time, financial resources, and cultural capital to follow the era's diet advice.[9] His diaries revolve around his efforts to promote his health and build his body through exercise and diet. Interestingly, he writes very little about his actual health problems. Based on a few entries, however, we can surmise that Rhoads likely suffered from neurasthenia, since he saw a "nervous expert" as soon as he arrived at the sanitarium.[10] Neurasthenia was regarded as a sickness of weak nerves and was a particularly common diagnosis among white elites in the decades around 1900.[11] Male neurasthenia was usually treated with a strict regimen of diet and exercise, and on these topics Rhoads wrote copiously. After swinging weighted clubs at the Young Men's Christian Association (YMCA) once or twice daily for several years, he started to exercise at home. Rhoads ordered clubs and rings and turned his family's home workshop into a gym, exercising sometimes as much as a few hours a day.[12] While his early diaries focus primarily on his exercises and only sometimes mention his food intake, diet started to play an increasingly important role after Rhoads's visits to Battle Creek in the years 1901 and 1902, and even more so between 1916 and 1918, when he struggled mightily with his diet.

In this chapter, I discuss these diaries in regard to questions of food, power, and agency. It is a risky endeavor to concentrate mainly on one source, a source that is also somewhat fragmentary.[13] However, Rhoads's diaries are an illuminating example of a very rare kind of source: one that helps us trace the everyday dietary practices of an individual around 1900. Rhoads's documentation of activities, food intake, and contemporary expertise allows us to understand his dietary practices in the context of the era's nutritional discourse and to locate his efforts in a broader white, middle-class engagement with healthy eating.

At first, I turn to the principles of diet promoted at Battle Creek Sanitarium and by nutritional science in the Progressive Era. Then, I focus more specifically on Rhoads and his practice of diary writing and explore two arguments concerning the nexus of food, power, and agency: first, I understand Rhoads's dieting as a technology of the self, which is in his case closely connected with the keeping of his diary as another technology of the self. Thus, both eating and writing are presented as practices by which Rhoads sought to shape himself as a self-responsible subject exerting agency. Second, my chapter complicates the notion of human agency by showing how it is enacted in networks of human and nonhuman actors.

"Hydropathic pudding is positively awful": Scientific eating in Battle Creek and elsewhere

When Rhoads is in Battle Creek, his rather short diary entries deal with his treatments, exercises, and sometimes his tiredness; letters he received from family members; recreational activities at the sanitarium; and most of all the weather.[14] Whereas Rhoads mentions his daily regimen of treatments (though often subsumed under "usual treatments"), it is particularly interesting that he rarely writes about the food served at the sanitarium. After all, a regulated diet was the cornerstone of therapy at Battle Creek, and it was one of the first things that new patients wrote about in their letters home.[15] For example, Louise C. Ketter of Marietta, Ohio, who spent about two months in the sanitarium in 1886, wrote to a friend, "As far as food is concerned, it is different from anything I ever got hold of." After describing the kind of cereals and fruits, vegetables and main dishes the sanitarium served for breakfast and dinner, she continued: "[F]or desserts they bring on some pretty fair dishes, some not fit to taste. Hydropathic pudding is positively awful. I tasted it and with difficulty swallowed it, old cheese it tasted of. … But you must remember that everything is hygienic."[16]

If Maxwell Rhoads disliked the hydropathic pudding, he did not entrust this information to his diary. Maybe it was because it was only by staying at the sanitarium that he became convinced of the enormous role that food played in gaining and maintaining health. Or maybe Rhoads did not mention the bill of fare at Battle Creek because he was already familiar with it and thus it did not come as a surprise. In any case, food was already a factor in his struggle for health before he came to the sanitarium. We know, for example, that he ordered "nut food" in early October 1898, shortly before he visited Battle Creek for the first time.[17] However, considering the rising number of food entries in his diary, it is clear that his interest in "hygienic" food piqued dramatically after his stay at Battle Creek. A few days after his first arrival at the sanitarium, Rhoads bought a copy of Ella Kellogg's famous cookbook *Science in the Kitchen*.[18] J. H. Kellogg's wife had collaborated with her husband to create the products and recipes that were used at Battle Creek, and she led a cooking school for the sanitarium's patients.[19] Over the course of more than 600 pages, she elaborated on "the science of dietetics, or what might be termed the hygiene of cookery."[20] Rhoads was probably delighted by the scientific rigor that characterized the cookbook as well as the treatment at the sanitarium. Two days after buying the book, he "ordered 100 lbs. of health food" from the sanitarium for $11.25.[21] During his second visit, he bought "20 bromose tablets" from one of the staff members.[22] Bromose was a product of nuts and predigested starch that was recommended to, among others, neurasthenic and dyspeptic patients.[23] Rhoads apparently liked and used these tablets since he bought another twenty-five of them only twelve days later.[24] On the last day of his second visit, he again ordered health foods at the sanitarium's so-called health bureau and had them delivered to his home in Anderson.[25] His diary gives the impression that Rhoads left Battle Creek very much convinced of the principles of "hygienic living." For instance, regarding a family friend, he noted in July 1900, "Saw Anna K[eltner]. She ... looks frail. Six months of hygienic living + proper exercise would do wonders for her."[26] But what did Ketter, Kellogg, and Rhoads mean when they talked about "hygienic living"?

"Hygienic" or "scientific eating" was one of the key principles of the sanitarium. Kellogg, influenced by food reformer Sylvester Graham, was obsessed with the dangers of eating the wrong kind of food, overeating, and "autointoxication." In keeping with his dietary convictions, he promised his patients to cure their sicknesses through the careful selection of foods and the total reformation of their eating habits.[27] In his numerous publications, he detailed the relationship between food and sicknesses like neurasthenia, dyspepsia, and various other conditions seen as dangerous to people's bodies and minds.[28] Hence, Kellogg belonged to the "new nutrition" movement that established in the late nineteenth-century United States a close connection between diet and science.[29] The momentum of this movement is vividly illustrated by the history of the Battle Creek Sanitarium. Founded as a convalescent home for Seventh Day Adventists in 1866, the institution changed when Kellogg became its director in 1876. The recently graduated medical doctor from a well-known Adventist family was hired to develop and expand the health institute. He opened it for patients of all denominations, called it a "sanitarium" to stress that it "served as a locale of both recovery *and* learning," and thereby fueled the change of diet advice from religious-oriented guidance to knowledge founded on modern scientific principles.[30] The magazine published by the institution also exemplifies this turn. Under the aegis of Kellogg, the journal changed its name from *The Health Reformer* to simply *Good Health*, and changed its content as well. The reformist, overtly spiritual tone gave way to "reports on German bacteriological research, articles on world-wide developments in surgery, nutrition and physiological chemistry." Thereby, as historian Gerald Carson writes, "the religious-medical-popular health movement brought forward a different kind of evidence."[31] This was indeed true when nutritional advice increasingly came with the authority of physicians, chemists, and other scientific experts.[32]

This new kind of evidence was powerfully persuasive for contemporaries. It fit well into the era's zeitgeist and was part of a plethora of social forces and rationales that shaped Progressive politics and personal practices. In an era of drastic social change and mass industrialization, urbanization, and immigration, many people believed in the power of scientific expertise to order an allegedly disordered society.[33] Nutritional knowledge and eating practices became part of the "regenerative enterprises," as the historian T. J. Jackson Lears has characterized this time in which personal health was increasingly and directly linked to public health and civilization's progress.[34] Progressives pressed for the reform of the individual as well as of society. More precisely, many people started to believe that individual reform could benefit society at large. Especially in the fields of nutrition and health, the connection between individual and social health seemed obvious. Moreover, at a time when fear of racial decline was widespread in white America, a healthy body stood for the possibility of social advancement, and eugenicists (and later euthenists) stressed the benefits of proper eating for individual bodies as well as for the "white race."[35] Next to direct references to racial advancement by nutrition experts who suggested, for example, that the eating of meat would greatly benefit a race, notions of dietary hygiene were highly symbolic.[36] For instance, Kellogg advocated a meat-free diet in order to keep one's blood free from toxins and "impurities."[37] In a time when the ultraracist "one-drop" rule was on the rise, it was not difficult to understand "pure blood" as a metaphor for racial purity.[38] This indicates that not only was the link between meat eating and racial progress highly controversial but, putting all other differences aside, it also shows that racial progress was among the main objectives of the food reformers. Kellogg's later project, the Race Betterment Foundation, vividly demonstrated the eugenic ethos of food reform in the Progressive Era.[39]

The biopolitical power of nutritional science can hardly be underestimated. Dietary knowledge proved especially powerful since it combined ideals of science, economic efficiency, and racial uplift.[40] Euthenics, a new "science of controllable environment" and a supplement to eugenics, aimed to ensure "efficient human beings [through increase of scientific knowledge]."[41] It was no accident that Kellogg also became an activist in the Health and Efficiency League, along with economist Irving Fisher and food reformer Horace Fletcher in 1909.[42] Food science and economic thought were closely connected. Home economist Ellen Richards, for instance, subtitled her treatise on the scientific optimization of living conditions with an epigraph from Fisher's *Report on National Vitality*: "The national annual unnecessary loss of capitalized net earnings is about $1,000,000,000."[43] This amount of money, lost by "preventable deaths," would add up, with the costs of illnesses, to "at least a billion and a half of preventable waste."[44] In this light, national health became a question of economics, and the discourse of diet and nutrition was a formidable yet inviting terrain for Progressive reform endeavors since it could vividly demonstrate the dangers of waste and sickness. With the normalization of health and the link between health and a proper diet increasingly established, healthy eating became a question of personal economy and racial progress. The close connection between "scientific" nutrition and an alleged increase in efficiency contributed to the era's obsession with fitness—of the body as well as of the mind. "Energy," Lears writes, became an "end in itself."[45] And this went hand in hand with a new emphasis on the malleability of bodies: in the decades around 1900, experts stressed the role of food in shaping and changing bodies, with effects ranging from weight loss to the euthenist notion of perfecting the race through proper nutrition.[46] When health became a scientific norm and merged paradigms of the economic, the social, and the political, having an able body became a powerful normative ideal. This "compulsory able-bodiedness," to borrow the queer theorist's Robert McRuer's term, prompted people to continuously strive for self-improvement, thus embodying the Progressive Era's impetus toward individual and collective regeneration and progress.[47]

However, it is important to note that the emphasis on a specific, expertly planned diet to improve health and fitness was basically a white, middle-class and, thus, exclusive ideal—symbolically as well as financially. As the earlier history of fasting and fat-reducing diets shows, dieting was associated with self-restraint and the masterful control of bodily impulses—abilities that were associated with the emerging white, manly middle-class and that figured to be crucial to their alleged superiority.[48] Moreover, choosing what to eat and eating special health foods was something one had to be able to afford. Rhoads spent a great deal of time, money, and effort on his exercise and diet. Ordering health foods, for instance, was not easy at that time. Being part of the upper middle class, his problem, though, was not so much a financial one as a logistical one. In late 1900, Rhoads tried for a while to place an order with Kellogg's Sanitas Food Company, but the company initially rejected his order on the basis that they only "sell on to wholesalers."[49] After eventually clearing this hurdle and successfully placing the order, Rhoads had to go to the freight depot almost every day for ten days to see whether his foods had arrived.[50] Until several years later, when a bourgeoning health foods market created the possibility for affluent customers to buy foods through a broad network of mail order catalogues and stores, purchasing these specialty goods required time and effort in addition to mere financial resources.[51] And in other respects, Rhoads and his family literally went to great distances for the sake of their health. In 1901, the family uprooted and moved to California (initially to San Diego and, in 1902, to La Jolla) so that Maxwell and Adaline would benefit from the healthier climate.[52]

Although arranging his life around becoming healthy was an elaborate endeavor for Rhoads, we can assume that his way of eating and organizing his life gave him a kind of pleasure. For example, on Thanksgiving Day 1899, the nineteen-year-old noted, "Today I partook of boiled wheat, nuttolene, whole wheat wafers + zwieback, grapes + an apple while the rest of the family dined on roast turkey, dressing, gravy, sweet potatoes, mashed potatoes, bread, oysters, cranberries, cellery [sic], olives, grapes, fruit cake + mince-pie [sic]." Rhoads's family enjoyed an abundant Thanksgiving dinner, while he ate different foods at a different time (at the sanitarium, the timing of meals was thought to be as important as the food eaten).[53] However, he did not complain about his bill of fare. On the contrary, he started that day's entry by announcing: "A lovely Thanksgiving day."[54]

While we already know that Rhoads ordered "health foods" from the sanitarium, entries like the above offer insight into the specific kinds of foods that he consumed. Rhoads regularly ate a range of the sanitarium's signature products like bromose, protose, nuttolene, granola, and granose.[55] These foods were distinctly branded "health food" inventions from the Kelloggs.[56] They were intended as substitutes for foodstuffs that Kellogg urged his patients to avoid. Nuttolene and protose, for instance, made from peanuts and wheat gluten, were designed to function as meat substitutes, while the purpose of bromose was to mimic the flavor and viscosity of milk.[57] Kellogg marketed other foods as particularly pure and digestible cereals. The famous Corn Flakes (which Kellogg created together with his brother Will) were only the most visible and profitable result of Kellogg's continuous efforts to produce the perfect Grahamite breakfast cereal. Already in 1877, Kellogg had invented granola, which he later advanced to granose, with the suffix "ose" stressing that the cereals were already predigested.[58] The increasingly successful Sanitas Nut Food Company that J. H. Kellogg owned together with his brother produced these foods.[59] In addition to the specialty foods company, the sanitarium was an economic success as well. It attracted a growing number of patients, who generally belonged to the middle and upper classes.[60] While it was not prohibitively expensive for many individuals to make a visit to Battle Creek (apparently, Rhoads paid $12 for his room for three and a half months; there were no additional costs for board and treatment), one had to have not only the money but also the time to stay at the sanitarium.[61] That predominantly the middle and upper classes were attracted to the health and economic benefits of scientific eating was already a contemporary verdict that linked a proper diet even more closely to social status.[62] However, it also safeguarded the economic success of Battle Creek and the health food industry in general.[63]

The success of Kellogg's enterprises demonstrated the possibility of capitalizing on people's longing for health and on the wholesale promises of "new nutrition." After all, Rhoads bought not only health food but also health expertise. He held subscriptions to the *Journal of Physical Culture* and *Good Health*, and he was a regular reader of the *Ladies' Home Journal* as well as other contemporary advice manuals on nutrition and fitness.[64] Moreover, Rhoads wrote to experts like Bernarr McFadden and later Otto Carqué for advice on his exercise and diet.[65] However, the power of health advice had its limits. Although Rhoads sought expertise and was obviously a fan of Battle Creek and its products, he did not "buy" everything Kellogg recommended. For instance, Rhoads was an eager visitor of so-called magnetic wells, drilled springs that were said to be magnetic and thus have curative power.[66] For a few years after 1900, he went to magnetic wells regularly, often once or twice a day, even on the day of his brother's funeral.[67] As early as 1876, Kellogg, however, had denounced those magnetic wells as "ingenious humbugs" that would "[dupe] [t]housands of people."[68] While we can assume that Rhoads knew of Kellogg's critique since he had spent so much time at Battle Creek, he clearly did not listen.

"Had very bad night. Also had ½ cake Hershey's almond chocolate": Eating and writing as technologies of the self

Until 1901 we only learn what Rhoads ate on special occasions. However, in the months and years following his visits to Battle Creek, he began describing his food intake in greater detail and increasingly tried to adhere to a stricter dietary regimen.

On February 8, 1901, for example, Rhoads embarked on a fasting cure, consuming only water to get rid of "a few slight temporary ailments."[69] Fasting was a common practice at that time, recommended to relieve digestive diseases and regarded as a manly exercise to demonstrate self-control and build a hardened body.[70] Just one day after Rhoads resolved to abstain from eating, however, he confessed in his diary, "I broke my fast and took two light meals on fruit and one on solid food."[71] He did not offer any further commentary on his fast breaking and did not attempt it again until one year later when he also persevered for only one day.[72] What started with these efforts, however, was a growing preoccupation with his dietary intake, a preoccupation that was fueled and reflected by the content and style of Rhoads's diary entries. Initially, Rhoads made his food intake part of a narrative, with entries such as, "I have just finished dinner, removed my apple peelings + two egg shells + put back in the refrigerator the remaining crab-apples, crackers, whole wheat bread, granola, crystal wheat + nut butter."[73] Soon, however, his entries consisted predominantly of bald facts: "Today my dinner consisted of watermelon, apples and peaches."[74] During the years that followed, Rhoads became a more precise documentarian of his diet. A typical entry from 1902 read, "For breakfast I ate a spoonful of grape-nuts, 1 bromose, 2 crisps, ½ piece of zwieback with nut b. + 1 ½ apples. For dinner (4:15) I ate 2 spoonfuls of grape-n[uts]. + 1 of granola ½ piece of zwieback with n[ut]b[utter] 2 oz. of granose flakes + small piece (about cu. in.) of protose [all: sic]."[75] Rhoads's dietary accounts suggest that he was following some kind of fruit and nut diet. The Kelloggs recommended this diet for the treatment of a range of ailments, including digestive problems and headaches that were oftentimes also associated with neurasthenia.[76] Thus, it is difficult to conclude whether Rhoads was still fighting off neurasthenia (or any other sickness) or whether he was trying to achieve another, maybe more general, dietary and bodily goal. In any case, Rhoads's preoccupation with what he ate became increasingly intense, and the assessment of his food intake grew more and more precise—one might say more "scientific." This becomes even clearer in his later diaries. Written between 1916 and 1918, the entries are a rich source of insight into Rhoads's daily struggles with food. In the meantime, Rhoads had become a dairy farmer, owning between eight and ten cows and selling their calves, milk, and cream.[77] In these years, Rhoads recorded his diet even more diligently than before. It was a daily topic, initially among other things, and later the sole content of his entries.

Rhoads's diaries allow us to grasp his eating and writing as technologies of subjectivation, that is, as practices of making and transforming his self.[78] Michel Foucault described such modes as "way[s] in which the individual establishes his relation to the rule and recognizes himself as obliged to put it into practice."[79] Subjectivation, thus, does not only mean to subject oneself to norms such as healthy dieting. It is through this subjection that an individual emerges as a self and attains agency. In Rhoads's diary, writing and eating emerge as practices that simultaneously confined and enabled and hence produced Rhoads as a dieting self.

To begin with the writing, in the late nineteenth century, journaling was among the central ideals and means of Victorian selfhood and progress. Advice givers recommended it especially for young people, girls as well as boys, to learn and document daily discipline and self-improvement.[80] Rhoads kept his journal as a practice of self-scrutiny, as the very first entry of 1916 makes clear. "Many entries in this book," he wrote, "to an outsider, would seem very trivial + useless of recording but I am keeping this diary mainly for purposes of comparison + reference in matters of health + business."[81] The reference to comparison suggests that he kept track of his diet not only by documenting it but also by comparing it to previous habits. And indeed, there is at least one entry that makes this process explicit. "Compare Mar 31 with 24th [sic]," he wrote on March 24, indicating that he had tried to improve his diet.[82] By writing, Rhoads assessed, compared, and thereby, made sense of his food intake and himself.

In addition to his writing, eating itself served as a technology of the self. It was no coincidence that Rhoads sought comparison at a time when food became comparable in a way that it had not been before. The classification of nutritional values such as protein, carbohydrates, and fat as well as the invention of the calorie in the late nineteenth century created the possibility of comparing different foodstuffs and the diets of different people and populations.[83] Although Rhoads did not explicitly refer to these categories, as we will see, he did classify certain foods as dairy and sugar and measured his portions precisely. Moreover, assessing his food intake as such allowed Rhoads to link his diet to his health and productivity. Although he rarely wrote directly about the condition of his health, some entries give a glimpse into his reasoning in this respect. Sometime during the night of March 24, 1918, he felt sick. He assumed that the "mid day [sic] luncheon" from earlier in the day was responsible for that.[84] And a few days later, he noted, "[b]ad headache nearly all night. I will try just a gill of hot water at noon instead of a whole cup."[85] In later years, when Rhoads had to get up early in the morning to milk the cows and make the rounds selling milk and cream, he related his ability to do that properly to the food he had in the morning or the day before: "I had to have big breakfast as I had a hard morning," he wrote for instance on April 3, 1918. His cows had gotten out of pasture, so he "had a lot of running to do."[86] And when he felt weak, like he did on April 14 of that year, he reacted by simply eating "a little more food" than usual.[87]

Rhoads assumed a causal link between diet, health, and his ability to work. This assumption reflected the increasingly widespread Progressive belief in the central promise of "scientific eating," namely, that the optimal food for body and mind could be precisely determined. Because of this assumption, health became a question of personal conduct, that is, of choosing the right things to eat. Hence, nutritional advice came with a powerful demand. It was accompanied by the expectation that individuals took responsibility for their health and chose their foods wisely. This was even more important since, as mentioned above, reformers understood individual health as contributing to or mirroring the condition of the race or the nation, making a close self-examination of diet and bodily fitness imperative. While a moral ideal of a self-culture already shaped mid-nineteenth-century understandings of Victorian manliness, it literally turned physical at the end of the century.[88] Diet and nutrition formed a discursive field where, in a Foucauldian perspective, the government of the population was closely intertwined with individual regulation—a regulation that was not coerced but acted upon voluntarily by the historical actors, often with pleasure.[89] Rhoads's pursuit of eating right points to the era's ideal of self-examination, comparison, and control in an effort to achieve truly efficient bodies and selves.

Rhoads apparently felt the need for advice when it came to questions of self-control. In April 1916, for instance, he noted that he had read *Your Will Power*, by Charles Godfrey Leland, a self-help treatise that promised to teach readers "How to Develop and Strengthen Will Power."[90] In June 1918, Rhoads wrote to the Emerson Institute of Efficiency, an institution that offered business consulting as well as courses in "personal efficiency" that promised to show participants how to optimize the efficiency of their "brain," "health," and "time."[91] In reading Rhoads's diary from late 1916 through early 1918, one gets the impression that he tried even more than before to control his diet and get better. In these later years, we find him eating different foods than previously. In the morning, he often drank a cup of chocolate, and biscuits as well as cake also turn up in his diet. Generally, every ounce of milk, every piece of zwieback, and every slice of cake found its way into his diary. And especially in regard to foods like cake (and milk to a lesser extent), he apparently was not pleased with his eating habits. One of the most striking changes between the two periods of diaries available is that Rhoads constantly worked on changing his eating habits in these later entries. Already in October 1916, Rhoads conceived the plan to " 'cut out' the pie and all confections + pastry for a few months." However, as a comment from a year later drily testifies, he had "failed to keep that resolution." Only a few days after he had made this diet plan in 1916, he listed cookies among other things in his diet report without commenting on it.[92] In February 1918, after he had been sick with a cold for a few weeks, he started to keep his diary again.[93] Maybe the sickness and the perceived need to begin documenting his food intake played a role in starting the diary again. In any case, diet and work took center stage in his entries from this point on, many of which consisted of mere stenographical notes like "bran + raisins, hygienic crax, . . ., cup cereal for breakfast. At 4 PM. boiled onion, 2 eggs + Krumbles, . . ., crax, nut b. Milked 6 cows, bottled milk [all: sic]."[94] On February 28, after he had eaten bran and dried fruits as well as different grain and milk dishes, he added (with a different pencil), "I will eat no more milk, meat, sugar, cream, candy or pastry of any kind for 60 days, not before May 1."[95] Being a dairy farmer, the promise to avoid milk and cream was an ambitious one. After three days of not recording his diet, he had milk for dinner (among other things) and moaned that he would "still feel . . . rotten with bronchitis + [a] bad cough." Although he did not comment on his milk intake on that day, he planned a rigorous diet for the next day. For breakfast and dinner, he intended to eat only "bran with figs, 2 hygienic crax, hot water." Moreover, he wanted to drink "at least 3 pts. hot [water] thru the day."[96] He did not do that. Along with eggs, granola, and zwieback, he also had cream and milk, without explicitly judging it. In the following days, he consumed sugar, cream, and milk, though he did not comment on it beyond documenting every ounce eaten. On March 10, he ate meat and cake, but added, "Today no milk no cream."[97]

What is particularly striking here is the ambivalence between Rhoads's plans and the documentation of his failure to achieve them. In reading the entries from early 1918, one gets the impression that the more he tried to avoid distinct foods, the more he ate of them and the more diligently he recorded this. The entry from March 11, for instance, is a good example of the dynamics of Rhoads's struggles to control his diet:

> Breakfast can of Campbells chicken gumbo, 6 pcs zwieback, butter on 2 of them, 1 ½ hyg[ienic] crax, dish peas.
>
> No milk, cream, sugar, pastry.
>
> Very rainy. Went to S[an] D[iego] at 7:30 + had treatment from Byars. Rested, then went to Angelus + got room for 1 ½ hours. Went to S. D. bank and fd 110.00 on acct. Cup coffee at Olsens (cream + sugar).
>
> Last night retired at 7, slept until 11:45. Not much after that. Coughed very little tho, last night.
>
> Dinner 4:30 to 6:30, 3 eggs with Krumbles, 5 pcs zwieback, 4 hyg. crax, dairy butter and nut b. large dish peas, later about a dozen little oatmeal cookies + 2 cups or more butter milk Rainy all day.
>
> 7:30 [with a different pencil]: No more milk, cream, butter, nuts, sugar, meat, pastry or condiments of any description until I have been back on both routes 10 days [all: sic].[98]

This entry is remarkable since Rhoads, after noting that he had not consumed dairy or sugar in the morning, broke his intent on the same day only to renew it mantra-like at the end of the day. Apparently, he felt bad about not following his diet plan and again promised himself to stick to it, only to continue his struggle anew. "[A] little dairy butter" was already on the diet list the next day. The day after that, Rhoads kicked it into high gear and had "3 or more cups milk, 2 cups hot chocolate, 8 little oatmeal cookies, 2 spoonfuls powdered chocolate!!!" A while later, he had more cookies and milk and commented, "I almost believe a man can get drunk on milk."[99] By referring to drunkenness in 1918 in the middle of the debate on prohibition, Rhoads convened the specters of indulgence, immorality, and social breakdown.[100] Perhaps this explains why, after his diet included meat, cream, milk, and cookies during the two days that followed, he noted apologetically, "Am trying the very heavy eating plan to get rid of this cold. If it doesn't work, will eat lightly again."[101] Apparently, it did not work. Rhoads continued to eat exactly what he was trying to avoid. When Rhoads visited San Diego, he usually went on a sort of cake frenzy. After his regular doctor's appointment and one or two hours of rest at Hotel Angelus, he went to a place called Olson's grill, had coffee (with cream and sugar) and most often "apple pie a la mode" as well as coffee cake and occasionally candy. After these indulgences, he sometimes bought a "Herscheys [sic] choc" cake or two.[102] After a few days like this, he confessed, "Failed to keep my agreement with myself, but will try again." And then he added, "Had very bad night last night, high fever for awhile + terribly sore in chest. Also had ½ cake Hersheys almond chocolate."[103]

Rhoads's struggles continued into April, and his records of his food intake remained a central feature of his diary. Surprisingly, Rhoads rarely commented on his apparent failures to keep his resolutions, and when he did, the comments were more offhand and prosaic than reproachful. However, these accounts of intents and failures present a strong contrast to the much more coherent narratives of eating right that Rhoads offered in his earlier diaries. He continued to make and renew his resolutions of better eating and likely believed that his health would benefit from increased dietary self-control. In short, a link between proper nutrition, will power and self-control shaped Rhoads's diary entries during this period far more than in the years between 1898 and 1902. They also portray healthy eating as a never-ending task, as a future-oriented practice aimed at achieving a fundamentally unachievable ideal. In the later years of diary writing, Rhoads, now in his mid-thirties, was still longing for betterment. In early February 1916, for example, after he came back from a walk, he noted with wistful determination, "Wish I would always feel as good as I did when I returned from that walk. I <u>will</u> some day."[104]

Besides documenting his ongoing dietary struggles, Rhoads's diaries reveal how the keeping of a journal allowed him to struggle in the first place, to conduct and assess himself and his diet, to make plans, to execute them or not, and to constantly try anew. Writing and eating emerge as corresponding and entangled technologies of the self that only superficially conflicted when Rhoads noted that he broke his fast or had cake again. Rhoads's dense documentation of his diet already served as a visible sign of an increased attention to the self. Perhaps Rhoads was able to exercise the necessary self-examination merely by recording what he ate day after day, including apple pie à la mode. By writing in his diary, Rhoads did the "diet work" necessary to perform self-examination and control. Thus his reports can be understood as part of his dietary conduct, of him exerting agency even in moments of struggle and failure. That is to say, the very act of keeping a journal allowed Rhoads to document and, perhaps even more importantly, to negotiate what eating right meant for him. This relation of control and failure becomes even more complex when we turn our attention to power and agency in the intricate networks of human and nonhuman actors.

The agency of apple pie à la mode

For Rhoads, food entailed the power to make him better, and he likely saw himself, as well as the foods he consumed, as the agents of this change. Taking a closer look at the difference these foods made, I now probe the question of how insightful an acknowledgment of the foodstuffs' agency is for the analysis of historical eating practices and the power embodied in them.

How can we understand the importance that these foods—or a distinct diet in general—held in Rhoads's life? From today's standpoint, some of his convictions with regard to the effects of foodstuffs seem rather odd, such as avoiding the consumption of water when he had a headache. But when dealing with a historical field as naturalized as body and diet history, it is particularly challenging to avoid judging from the present-day point of view whether it was a sound and effective practice or sheer belief. Terms like "beliefs" and "convictions" (that I have used up to now with regard to Rhoads) do not help us either. They imply that the reality could have been different. In order to understand historical diet practices, however, looking for the reality behind people's beliefs misses the mark because this approach bends our view from these practices and the ways contemporary knowledge emerged and was stabilized. Therefore, how can we inquire into the difference that foodstuffs make without assuming either an ahistorical impact of certain foods or an illusionary faith of people, seduced by the food industry's false promises?

One possible analytical tool to deal with this epistemological problem is Bruno Latour's concept of the *faitiche* (*factish* in the English translation) that offers an alternative to the dichotomy of fact and belief. The neologism *faitiche* combines "fact" (*fait*) and "fetish" (*fétiche*) and refers to the impossibility of distinguishing between these two types. A factual objectivity is as fabricated as beliefs, Latour suggests, and vice versa. Beliefs are no less real—or autonomous, as he would say. According to Latour, the need to choose between fact and fetish is a problematic heritage of modernity and represents an inappropriate dichotomy for describing and analyzing the assemblage of the social.[105] *Faitiches*, alternatively, are "types of action that do not fall into the comminatory choice between fact and belief."[106] However, as Latour warns, this does not mean that everything is "illusion, storytelling and make believe." Rather, it is necessary to account for the immense autonomy and agency of *faitiches*.[107]

Following Latour's suggestion, it is key to analyze where things "make a difference in the course of some other agent's action," where they make others act, where they "authorize, allow, afford, encourage, permit, suggest, influence, block, render possible, forbid" the actions of others.[108] When things or people "make" other people or things "do" something, Latour speaks of actors.[109] Rhoads's diary, for instance, is such an actor. It made a crucial difference in his struggles for health by allowing and encouraging his dietary accounting. With the explicit inclusion of nonhuman actors, Latour disconnects agency from the intent of a strong-willed human being.[110] Seen from this perspective, there is no human agency that masterfully governs things and events, and the question of Rhoads's control and failure becomes increasingly complex. The apple pie à la mode and its sweet seductive force provide another good example of this dynamic. Looking closer at its agency, the pull it had with Rhoads, adds an additional layer to the analysis of his struggles for healthy eating that focuses on the "vital force" of matter.[111]

Even in liberal ideals of self-control, the notion of human agency and will is more complicated than it often seems, as Jane Bennett points out.[112] If we understand Rhoads's consumption of apple pie à la mode in a somewhat traditional sense as a repeated failure to control his diet, we also acknowledge another agent's force, another agent's ability to break the will of Rhoads's dieting self, to seduce him into eating the warm apple pie and cool ice cream, whether this agent be appetite, the stomach, or any other part of what is conceived of as Rhoads's body or self. This interpretation is based on the idea of body and mind as distinct entities, with the ideal of the mind controlling the body. In contrast to that, taking into account the agency of matter can move not only beyond the notion of a body/mind split but also beyond the sole focus on the agency of the self or of Rhoads as a human. Instead, it highlights the networks that Rhoads was part of. What could this mean in regard to the apple pie?

First of all, the apple pie à la mode obviously affected Rhoads. It animated him to eat it, and although he did not comment on eating the pie, we know that it made a difference. It changed the way Rhoads felt about his diet and his body, and at the very least it made him promise not to eat cake again. In Latour's terms, the apple pie fabricated Rhoads. It fabricated him as a dieter by shaping his dietary practices, but it fabricated him also by affecting his body. The apple pie literally acted through Rhoads by being eaten and becoming part of him. "[Food] enters into what we become," Bennett writes, and refers to the transformative "activity of metabolization, whereby the outside and inside mingle and recombine," blurring the boundaries between inside and outside as well as those between bodies.[113]

Moreover, by becoming part of Rhoads's body, the apple pie joined yet another complex actor network by which it was affected itself. It was brought to his mouth, chopped up by his teeth, swallowed, and digested, and thus became part of an assemblage of bowels, fluids, and cultural techniques. If the apple pie did help animate these activities, how much sense does it make to look exclusively for the intent of a human being in this event?[114] Of course, this is not to say that the apple pie is the only or even the determining actor at play. This interpretation does not mean to rob Rhoads of all intent but rather to understand this intent as only part of the agentic network. As Bennett stresses, and as my analysis of his dietary and writing practices showed, "it is also possible to say something about the kind of striving that may be exercised by a human within the assemblage."[115] However, it should already be clear why we cannot stop short by talking only about Rhoads's beliefs or convictions. By pointing to the agency of things, Latour stresses the performativity of actions and events: the fabrication of things invests them with stability, but it does not make them predictable or even controllable. Action always leads to surprises, he stresses: "[W]henever we make something *we* are not in command, we are slightly *overtaken* by the action."[116] Rhoads's intentions, as well as the apple pie, are only two actors in an actor network consisting of others, like the cake display and the waiter, or if one wants to be more precise, a hand, a table, a fork, a stomach, and enzymes, bringing forth something that is beyond the control of any one of them.

If we broaden the scene of the apple pie, different, overlapping assemblages of Rhoads's eating and writing become visible. In addition to understanding the materiality of the diary as enabling Rhoads to record his diet, writing and eating emerge as different assemblages of human and nonhuman actors: desk, pen, diary, hand, writer; and food, fork, mouth, eater. Taking into account this diverse enactment of agency and the way foods acted through Rhoads allows us to revisit the question of Rhoads's dietary struggles. From this perspective, the servings of apple pie à la mode (as well as the pastries, milk, and other things he tried to avoid) were not setbacks but the conditions of Rhoads's endeavor. He needed the cake for this. Without its temptation, there would be no meaning in dieting, no goal of "hygienic" eating. The cake enabled Rhoads to work on himself, to demonstrate this work, and to continue his striving. This moves us beyond narratives of failure to the performative power of agentic networks. It complicates the ideal of human (corporeal) agency—or the "fiction of the [autonomous and self-controlled] bourgeois I"—without portraying selves as mere victims of bodily or "outside" forces but rather as only one among a multitude of different actors.[117] Rhoads's agency becomes more complicated and visible as an agentic assemblage itself. This has consequences not only for understanding his relationship to food and food's impact on his life. It also critically questions the ideal of corporeal control and improvement. As Bennett argues, it "resist[s] a politics of blame,"[118] and thus, sheds new light on historical as well as contemporary practices of eating "right."

Notes

This chapter was written in the context of the research project "The Eating Self. A History of the Political in the United States from the 19th to the 21st century" (funded by the Thyssen Foundation). I am grateful to Juergen Martschukat and Bryant Simon, Silvan Niedermeier and Oliver Schmerbauch as well as the other contributors to this volume for their comments on earlier versions of this chapter.

Roland Barthes," Pour une psycho-sociologie de l'alimentation contemporaine," *Annales: Économies, Sociétés, Civilisations* 16, no. 5 (1961): 977–86. Cited here is the English version, "Toward a Psychosociology of Contemporary Food Consumption," in *Food and Culture: A Reader*, ed. Carole Counihan and Penny Van Esterik (1997; New York: Routledge, 2008), 33.

1 Diary of Roscoe Maxwell Rhoads, 1897–1898 (December 29, 1898), Papers of Horace Emerson Rhoads, Huntington Library, San Marino, CA.

2 Finding Aid for Papers of Horace Emerson Rhoads, 1886–1941, available online: Huntington Digital Library, accessed October 30, 2014, http://cdm16003.contentdm.oclc.org/cdm/singleitem/collection/p15150coll1/id/2602/rec/1.

3 Hillel Schwartz, *Never Satisfied: A Cultural History of Diets, Fantasies, and Fat* (New York: Anchor Books, 1986), 186.

4 Diaries of Roscoe Maxwell Rhoads, 1897–1898, 1899–1900, 1901–1902, 1916–1918, all: Papers of Horace Emerson Rhoads.

5 Gail Bederman, *Manliness & Civilization: A Cultural History of Gender and Race in the United States, 1880–1917* (Chicago and London: University of Chicago Press, 1995); R. Marie Griffith, *Born Again Bodies: Flesh and Spirit in American Christianity* (Berkeley: University of California Press, 2004); Jürgen Martschukat, "'The Necessity for Better Bodies to Perpetuate Our Institutions, Insure a Higher Development of the Individual, and Advance the Conditions of the Race': Physical Culture and the Formation of the Self in the Late Nineteenth and Early Twentieth Century USA," *Journal of Historical Sociology* 24, no. 4 (2011): 472–93; Nina Mackert, "'I want to be a fat man / and with the fat men stand'—U.S.-Amerikanische Fat Men's Clubs und die Bedeutungen von Körperfett in den Dekaden um 1900," *Body Politics* 3 (2014): 215–43.

6 Jackson Lears, *Rebirth of a Nation: The Making of Modern America, 1877–1920* (New York: Harper Collins, 2009).

7 Schwartz, *Never Satisfied*; Harvey A. Levenstein, *Revolution at the Table: The Transformation of the American Diet* (Berkeley: University of California Press, [1988] 2003); Helen Zoe Veit, *Modern Food, Moral Food: Self-Control,*

Science, and the Rise of Modern American Eating in the Early Twentieth Century (Chapel Hill: University of North Carolina Press, 2013); Charlotte Biltekoff, *Eating Right in America: The Cultural Politics of Food and Health* (Durham, NC: Duke University Press, 2013).

8 An exception here is Veit's inspiring analysis of personal letters to the US Food Administration (Veit, *Modern Food*).

9 Their sixth child, Horace, became a newspaper publisher, politician, and later the founder of the San Diego Athletic Club. His brother's diary is part of Horace's papers at the Huntington Library in San Marino, CA.

10 Diary of Roscoe Maxwell Rhoads, 1897–1898 (October 18, 1898).

11 On neurasthenia, see Tom Lutz, *American Nervousness, 1903: An Anecdotal History* (Ithaca, NY: Cornell University Press, 1991); Bederman, *Manliness & Civilization*; David Schuster, *Neurasthenic Nation: America's Search for Health, Happiness, and Comfort, 1869–1920* (New Brunswick, NJ: Rutgers University Press, 2011).

12 See, for example, Diary of Roscoe Maxwell Rhoads, 1897–1898 (September 28, 1898); Diary of Roscoe Maxwell Rhoads, 1899–1900 (July 9/17/25/30, September 2, 1899); Diary of Roscoe Maxwell Rhoads, 1900–1901 (March 28, 1901).

13 Unfortunately, the records do not include diaries for the years 1903–1915, leaving us only to speculate as to what exactly he did (and ate) in those years.

14 Diary of Roscoe Maxwell Rhoads, 1897–1898 (October 18-November 1, 1898, December 28–31); Diary of Roscoe Maxwell Rhoads, 1899–1900 (January 1–April 10, 1899, August 19, 1899). Such a way of journal keeping was quite common and was often recommended by advice givers, see Jane H. Hunter, "Inscribing the Self in the Heart of the Family: Diaries and Girlhood in Late-Victorian America," *American Quarterly* 44, no. 1 (1992): 51–81, here 54–8.

15 Cf. John Harvey Kellogg, *The Battle Creek Sanitarium System: History, Organization, Methods* (Battle Creek, MI: Gage Printing Co., 1908); Schwartz, *Never Satisfied*, 185–7; Adam D. Shprintzen, *The Vegetarian Crusade: The Rise of an American Reform Movement, 1817–1921* (Chapel Hill: University of North Carolina Press, 2013), 124.

16 Louise C. Ketter to Elizabeth G. Stimson, March 7, 1886, Papers of Elizabeth Gillet Stimson Corwin, 1886–1943, Schlesinger Library, Harvard University, Cambridge, MA.

17 Diary of Roscoe Maxwell Rhoads, 1897–1898 (October 10, 1898).

18 Ibid. (October 26, 1898); Ella Eaton Kellogg, *Science in the Kitchen: A Scientific Treatise on Food Substances and Their Dietetic Properties, Together with a Practical Explanation of the Principles of Healthful Cookery, and a Large Number of Original, Palatable, and Wholesome Recipes* (Chicago: Modern Medicine Publishing Co., 1893).

19 Shprintzen, *Vegetarian Crusade*, 124f.

20 Kellogg, *Science in the Kitchen*, 3.

21 Diary of Roscoe Maxwell Rhoads, 1897–1898 (October 28, 1898).

22 Diary of Roscoe Maxwell Rhoads, 1899–1900 (January 23, 1899).

23 Cf. John Harvey Kellogg, *The Stomach: Its Disorders, and How to Cure Them* (Battle Creek, MI: Modern Medicine Pub. Co., 1896); Kellogg, *Science in the Kitchen*, 435–6.

24 Diary of Roscoe Maxwell Rhoads, 1899–1900 (February 4, 1899).

25 Ibid. (April 9 and April 17, 1899).

26 Ibid. (July 18, 1900).

27 Gerald Carson, *Cornflake Crusade* (New York and Toronto: Rinehart, 1957), 57; Schwartz, *Never Satisfied*, 183ff.; Harvey Levenstein, *Fear of Food: A History of Why We Worry about What We Eat* (Chicago: University of Chicago Press, 2012), chap. 3.

28 See, for instance, J. H. Kellogg, *The Household Manual of Hygiene, Food and Diet, Common Diseases, Accidents and Emergencies, and Useful Hints and Recipes* (Battle Creek, MI: The Office of the Health Reformer, 1877); Kellogg, *The Stomach;* J. H. Kellogg, *The New Dietetics: What to Eat and How: A Guide to Scientific Feeding in Health and Disease* (Battle Creek, MI: Modern Medicine Pub. Co., 1921).

29 Levenstein, *Revolution at the Table*, chapter 6.

30 Shprintzen, *Vegetarian Crusade*, 119–21 (quote on 121, emphasis in original). On the history of the sanitarium, see ibid., chapter 5; Carson, *Cornflake Crusade*.

31 Carson, *Cornflake Crusade*, 76f.

32 R. Marie Griffith has argued that this was by no means a process of secularization. On the contrary, the "new" knowledge was fraught with protestant ideals (Griffith, *Born Again Bodies*, 70f.).

33 Robert H. Wiebe, *The Search for Order, 1877–1920* (New York: Hill and Wang, 1967); Lears, *Rebirth of a Nation*.

34 Lears, *Rebirth of a Nation*, 4.

35 Ibid., chap. 3; Biltekoff, *Eating Right*, 28f.; Veit, *Modern Food*, chap. 5. Cf., for example, Ellen H. Richards, *The Cost of Food: A Study in Dietaries* (New York: John Wiley and Sons, 1901); Ellen H. Richards, *Euthenics: The Science of Controllable Environment*, 2nd ed. (Boston: Whitcomb & Barrows, [1910] 1912).

36 Cf., for instance, Sir James Crichton-Brown [sic], "Parsimony in Nutrition," *New York Times*, August 23, 1908: SM8. On euthenics and food, see Veit, *Modern Food*, chap. 5.

37 Shprintzen, *Vegetarian Crusade*, 124.

38 On the one-drop rule, see James Davis, *Who Is Black? One Nation's Definition*, 2nd ed. (University Park: Pennsylvania State Univ. Press, [1991] 2002).

39 Shprintzen, *Vegetarian Crusade*, 144.

40 See also Nina Mackert, "Feeding Productive Bodies: Calories, Nutritional Values and Ability in Progressive Era US," in *Histories of Productivity:*

Genealogical Perspectives on the Body and Modern Economy, ed. Peter-Paul Bänziger and Mischa Suter (London: Routledge 2016), 117–135.

41 Richards, *Euthenics*, vii.

42 Schwartz, *Never Satisfied*, 186; James C. Whorton, *Crusaders for Fitness: The History of American Health Reformers* (Princeton, NJ: Princeton University Press, 1982), 195.

43 Irving Fisher, *Report on National Vitality: Its Waste and Conservation* (Washington, DC: Government Printing Office, 1909), quoted in: Richards, *Euthenics*, title.

44 Fisher, *Report on National Vitality*, 120

45 Lears, *Rebirth of a Nation*, 27.

46 Katharina Vester, "Regime Change: Gender, Class, and the Invention of Dieting in Post-Bellum America," *Journal of Social History* 44, no. 1 (2010): 39–70; Veit, *Modern Food*, chapter 5.

47 Robert McRuer, *Crip Theory: Cultural Signs of Queerness and Disability* (New York and London: New York University Press, 2006), in particular 1–32. See also Mackert, "Feeding Productive Bodies."

48 Vester, "Regime Change"; R. Marie Griffith, "Apostles of Abstinence: Fasting and Masculinity during the Progressive Era," *American Quarterly* 52, no. 4 (2000): 599–638; Bederman, *Manliness & Civilization*.

49 Diary of Roscoe Maxwell Rhoads, 1900–1901 (October 30–November 7, 1900).

50 Ibid. (November 6–November 17, 1900).

51 Cf. Sphrintzen, *Vegetarian Crusade*, 130.

52 Cf., for instance, Diary of Roscoe Maxwell Rhoads, 1900–1901 (August 13ff., 1901). See also Finding Aid for Rhoads Papers, 3.

53 Ketter to Stimson, March 7, 1886.

54 Diary of Roscoe Maxwell Rhoads, 1899–1900 (November 30, 1899). See also similar entries in the following years (Diary of Roscoe Maxwell Rhoads, 1900–1901 [November 29, 1900; November 28, 1901]).

55 See, for instance, Diary of Roscoe Maxwell Rhoads, 1899–1900 (January 23, February 4, 1899), Diary of Roscoe Maxwell Rhoads, 1900–1901 (November 29, 1900; March 29, November 24/28, 1901), Diary of Roscoe Maxwell Rhoads, 1901–1902 (February 20, 1902).

56 Cf. Kellogg, *The Stomach*, 240f.

57 Carson, *Cornflake Crusade*, 108, 115; Shprintzen, *Vegetarian Crusade*, 131.

58 Carson, *Cornflake Crusade*, 124; Schwartz, *Never Satisfied*, 184, 186.

59 Shprintzen, *Vegetarian Crusade*, 130.

60 Schwartz, *Never Satisfied*, 186; Shprintzen, *Vegetarian Crusade*, 140.

61 Diary of Roscoe Maxwell Rhoads, 1897–1898 (December 28, 1898); Shprintzen, *Vegetarian Crusade*, 141 and 233. The average income of working-class families around that time was between eight and eighteen dollars a week, as a dietary study from 1896–97 indicates: Wilbur O.

Atwater and A. P. Bryant, *Dietary Studies in New York City in 1896 and 1897. Bulletin no. 116 of the US Department of Agriculture* (Washington, DC: Government Printing Office 1902).

62 Because the working class was regarded as indifferent to knowledge of healthy eating, one could perform class distinction even by talking about it (Cf. Levenstein, *Revolution at the Table*, especially chap. 4 and chap. 6; Biltekoff, *Eating Right*, chap. 2).

63 Shprintzen, *Vegetarian Crusade*, 130–4.

64 Cf., for instance, Diary of Roscoe Maxwell Rhoads, 1900–1901 (August 15, 1901); Diary of Roscoe Maxwell Rhoads, 1901–1902 (February 11–12, 1902).

65 Diary of Roscoe Maxwell Rhoads, 1900–1901 (May 15, 1901), Diary of Roscoe Maxwell Rhoads, 1916–1918 (January 4 and 16, 1916). On Macfadden, see Griffith, "Apostles of Abstinence." Carqué was a health food producer in the Los Angeles area who also wrote books on this topic. Otto Carqué, *The Foundation of All Reform: A Guide to Health, Wealth and Freedom: A Popular Treatise on the Diet Question* (Chicago: Kosmos Publishing, 1904). On Carqué, see William Shurtleff and Akiko Aoyagi, *History of Seventh-day Adventist Work with Soyfoods, Vegetarianism, Meat Alternatives, Wheat Gluten, Dietary Fiber and Peanut Butter (1863–2013): Extensively Annotated Bibliography and Sourcebook* (Lafayette, CA: Soyinfo Center, 2014), 1184.

66 Stiles Kennedy, *The Magnetic and Mineral Springs of Michigan, to Which is Prefixed an Essay on the Climate of Michigan* (Wilmington: James and Webb, 1872).

67 Cf., for example, Diary of Roscoe Maxwell Rhoads, 1897–1898 (September 26-October 4, 1898), Diary of Roscoe Maxwell Rhoads, 1899–1900 (August 18, 1899; July 9, 1900)

68 John Harvey Kellogg, *The Uses of Water in Health and Disease: A Practical Treatise on the Bath, Its History and Uses* (Battle Creek, MI: Office of the Health Reformer, 1876), 14.

69 Diary of Roscoe Maxwell Rhoads, 1901–1902 (February 8, 1901).

70 Kellogg, *The Stomach*, 167. The "symbolic repertoire" of fasting included, as historian R. Marie Griffith has shown, performances of manliness and masculinity, eugenic and capitalist understandings of health, bodily purity, and strength but also an emphasis on the pleasures of self-control. Griffith, "Apostles of Abstinence."

71 Diary of Roscoe Maxwell Rhoads, 1900–1901 (February 9, 1901).

72 Ibid. (February 15 and 16, 1901).

73 Ibid. (March 29, 1901). That Rhoads had access to a refrigerator is significant since home refrigerators were not common yet. Cf. Katherine Leonard Turner, *How the Other Half Ate: A History of Working-Class Meals at the Turn of the Century* (Berkeley: University of California Press, 2014), 32–3 and 59.

74 Diary of Roscoe Maxwell Rhoads, 1900–1901 (August 16, 1901).

75 Ibid., 1901–1902 (February 20, 1902). Grape-nuts, a breakfast cereal, were invented and marketed by Charles W. Post, a former patient and later competitor of Kellogg. Carson, *Cornflake Crusade*, 155f.

76 Kellogg, *Science in the Kitchen*, 435–6 and 441–4; Kellogg, *The Stomach*, 257.

77 Diary of Roscoe Maxwell Rhoads, 1916–1918. Before, Rhoads obviously did not have to do wage work. We do not know if he now needed to do it or if he did this for other reasons. He still lived with or close to his parents in La Jolla, California, and his brother Horace worked as manager of the *San Francisco Daily News* (Finding Aid for Rhoads Papers, 3).

78 Michel Foucault, "Technologies of the Self," in *Technologies of the Self: A Seminar With Michel Foucault*, ed. Luther H. Martin, Huck Gutman, and Patrick H. Hutton (Amherst: University of Massachusetts Press, 1988), 16–49.

79 Cf. Michel Foucault, *The History of Sexuality, vol. 2, The Use of Pleasure* (New York: Vintage Books, [1984] 1990), 10. See also Hunter, "Inscribing the Self," 52.

80 Using the examples of girls' diaries, Jane Hunter shows that such goals of self-improvement were not only the ideals of experts but also "made their way into girls' own self-expectations." Hunter, "Inscribing the Self," 54–60. Cf. also W. S. Jerome, "How to Keep a Journal," *St. Nicholas* 5 (October 1878), 789.

81 Diary of Roscoe Maxwell Rhoads, 1916–1918 (January 1, 1916).

82 Ibid., 1916–1918 (March 31, 1918).

83 Nick Cullather, "The Foreign Policy of the Calorie," *American Historical Review* 112, no. 2 (2007): 337–64, especially 340–7; Veit, *Modern Food*, 45; Mackert, Feeding Productive Bodies.

84 Diary of Roscoe Maxwell Rhoads, 1916–1918 (March 25, 1918).

85 Ibid. (March 29, 1918).

86 Ibid. (April 3, 1918).

87 Ibid. (April 14, 1918).

88 On diaries as technologies of the self for mid-nineteenth-century white middle-class men, see Thomas Augst, *The Clerk's Tale: Young Men and Moral Life in Nineteenth-Century America* (Chicago: University of Chicago Press, 2003).

89 Michel Foucault, *The History of Sexuality*, vol. 1, *An Introduction* (New York: Pantheon Books, [1976] 1978); Katharina Vester, *A Taste of Power: Food and American Identities* (Berkeley: University of California Press, 2015), 6; Veit, *Modern Food.*

90 Diary of Roscoe Maxwell Rhoads, 1916–1918 (April 2, 1916); Charles Godfrey Leland, *Your Will Power, Also Called The Mystic Will, Or How to Develop and Strengthen Will Power, Memory, or Any Other Faculty or Attribute of the Mind, by an Easy Process* (London: L. N. Fowler Co., 1918).

91 Diary of Roscoe Maxwell Rhoads, 1916–1918 (June 21, 1918); advertisement of the institute in: *Magazine of Business* 32 (1917): 837. Cf. also Emerson Institute of Efficiency, Indiana & Ohio Division, ed., *Possible Leaks and Losses in Manufacturing* (Marion, IN: R. E. Palmer, 1918).

92 Diary of Roscoe Maxwell Rhoads, 1916–1918 (October 22, 1916 [October 25, 1917, on the same page] and October 26, 1916).

93 In 1917, Rhoads wrote only very sparingly, we can only speculate why that was the case: Did everything go so well that he did not feel the need for recording his food intake and work?

94 Diary of Roscoe Maxwell Rhoads, 1916–1918 (February 22, 1918). "Hygienic crackers" were a product of the Hygienic Health Food Co., advertised as easily digestible food for people suffering from constipation, dyspepsia, and indigestion. US Department of Agriculture, "Notice of Judgement No. 1265: Alleged Misbranding of Grant's Hygienic Crackers, "issued February 24, 1912, available online: US National Library of Medicine, accessed November 1, 2014, http://archive.nlm.nih.gov/fdanj/handle/123456789/41322. "Krumbles" were another cereal product by Kellogg.

95 Diary of Roscoe Maxwell Rhoads, 1916–1918 (February 28, 1918).

96 Ibid. (March 4, 1918).

97 Ibid. (March 5–10, 1918).

98 Diary of Roscoe Maxwell Rhoads, 1916–1918 (March 11, 1918). We do not know why Rhoads had this appointment with Dr. Byars and what happened there exactly. However, he already went there in 1916, and it was a regular appointment in 1918, when Rhoads went to San Diego more than once a week for a while to get treated (cf., for instance, ibid. [January 10, 1916; March 18, 21, 25, and 30, April 2, 5, and 12, 1918]). It is unclear to the author what Rhoads referred to by "back on both routes."

99 Ibid. (March 13, 1918).

100 On temperance movement and prohibition, see Daniel Okrent, *Last Call: The Rise and Fall of Prohibition* (New York: Simon and Schuster, 2010).

101 Ibid. (March 15, 1918).

102 Cf. ibid. (March 15, 18, and 25, April 5 and 12, 1918).

103 Ibid. (March 19, 1918).

104 Ibid. (February 8, 1916); underlining in original.

105 Bruno Latour, *Pandora's Hope: Essays on the Reality of Science Studies* (Cambridge, MA: Harvard University Press, 1999), especially chap. 9.

106 Ibid., 316.

107 Ibid., 275.

108 Bruno Latour, *Reassembling the Social: An Introduction to Actor-Network-Theory* (Oxford: Oxford University Press, 2005), 71f.

109 Latour, *Pandora's Hope*, 288 and 313.

110 Latour, *Reassembling the Social*, 71.

111 Jane Bennett, *Vibrant Matter: A Political Ecology of Things* (Durham, NC: Duke University Press, 2010), 47.

112 Ibid., 28–9.

113 Bennett, *Vibrant Matter*, 49–51.

114 On human bodies as assemblages/actor networks, see ibid., 23 and 40.

115 Ibid., 38.

116 Latour, *Pandora's Hope*, 281, emphasis in original.

117 Theodor Adorno, quoted in Bennett, 16. See also the articles in the special issue, "Fat Agency," *Body Politics* 5 (2015).

118 Bennett, *Vibrant Matter*, 38.

6

"What diet can do": Running and eating right in 1970s America

Jürgen Martschukat

Everyone who is born holds dual citizenship, in the kingdom of the well and in the kingdom of the sick. Although we all prefer to use only the good passport, sooner or later each of us is obliged, at least for a spell, to identify ourselves as citizens of that other place.

SUSAN SONTAG, 1978[1]

Introduction

When in January 1978, Susan Sontag published her biting critique of the meaning of illness in America, Americans had been enmeshed in a new fitness craze for about a decade. While, as Sontag argued, 1970s America saw illness, particularly cancer, as a sign of resignation and of a bad attitude toward life and the self, fitness embodied power, agency, and a life-affirming attitude. Fitness meant not only a state of well-being but also, and perhaps more importantly, the practices and means employed to achieve that well-being, and Americans were more eager than ever to work actively toward obtaining and maintaining a passport to "the kingdom of the well." Americans were "shaping up," as a *Time Magazine* cover announced in November 1981. Representations of fit selves showed that the fit body of the 1970s and 1980s was not seen as the product of a disciplinary regime imposing its power and rules upon its citizens (as, for instance, a society mobilizing for wartime), but as the literal, physical embodiment of a new neoliberalism.[2] This was a society and culture based on its citizens' will to govern and take good care of themselves, thereby augmenting their ability to pursue happiness and strive for self-fulfillment and success in a social and political system defined by individualism and competition.

In the words of novelist and public intellectual Tom Wolfe, the understanding that individual self-fulfillment was the core purpose of human existence was a hallmark of American society and culture in the 1970s. In a widely read article in *New York Magazine*, Wolfe portrayed the 1970s as the "ME decade" (with "ME" intentionally capitalized for emphasis), in which self-fulfillment was more than ever at the center of American existence. At the same time, individuals themselves were held responsible for achieving happiness and self-fulfillment, and as Wolfe pointed out, the success or failure of their efforts was more than ever viewed as a function of corporeal perfection.[3] Millions of Americans were obsessed with their bodies and their fitness, which had become signifiers of their health and ability to function properly as citizens of a liberal society. The pursuit of happiness was being transformed into America's new civil religion, the pursuit of fitness.

Workouts were executed with a vigor and devotion that bordered on religious zeal, and particularly runners, daily growing in numbers, felt the inclination to share their personal testimonies with others of how they had been saved from a life of laziness, alcohol, fatty food, and physical decay. "I have abandoned the non-running world," was a typical statement found in a variety of magazines at the time. As one runner confessed in a letter to fitness apostle Kenneth Cooper, "I was in such bad shape, I weighed 247 pounds and my heart would beat like a drum when I got up from my chair to go to the refrigerator."[4]

The following chapter shows how, in 1970s America, a fit body became a powerful signifier of success and civic worth in a neoliberal society. This chapter focuses on the running culture, as running became the most iconic form of 1970s exercise with its major purpose of improving one's physical fitness. Yet the following pages do not discuss training manuals, patterns, and practices, but rather first and foremost depict the role that food acquired in America's pursuit of fitness through running. As an analysis of *Runner's World*—the Bible of US running publications—shows, the significance of eating and drinking right steadily increased among America's community of runners as well as in the burgeoning running consumer culture. As I demonstrate, the early 1970s idea of how food and fitness interact was still vague. Yet at the end of the decade, runners had no doubt about the power of energy drinks, such as Body Punch, or the fact that eating right (in their everyday life and particularly before races) made a difference in their efforts to optimize themselves and their fitness.

Thinking about the relation between running and fitness in neoliberal culture prompts us to reframe the concept of power and agency. As a concept, agency has been shaped in postcolonial studies[5] and in the history of everyday life, and here in particular by the thought and writing of historian Alf Lüdtke.[6] Here, agency denotes a combination of self-reliance, self-will, and self-respect among historical actors who somehow manage to reappropriate alienated and seemingly overpowering discourses, social relations, structures, and processes, which had previously appeared to be beyond their control. By means of their agency, marginalized historical actors use cultural resources as well as economic and political structures in a transformative way and thereby create a grammar different from existing hegemonic patterns.

Yet in neoliberal society, agency does not necessarily possess the power to liberate, since actively shaping one's life and maximizing one's personal potential has become an obligation. Liberalism is built on the premise that citizens use their freedom reasonably and efficiently, which proves their ability and productivity as members of a free society. Liberal societies are based on the concept of "governing through freedom,"[7] with government understood as a wide array of forces inciting individuals to action by nudging them to prove their ability to self-govern, optimize their lives, and make themselves citizens of the kingdom of the well[8] by virtue of their reason, self-control, and agency. Therefore, agency in a neoliberal order is not a means of resistance or withdrawal but rather one of compliance with the premises of social and political power and their demands.

If we add food to this equation and consider the relationships among running, fitness, and food in neoliberal culture, then we must reexamine the concepts of power and agency at an even more fundamental level. If we understand, with a nod to Bruno Latour, the social as a network of associations, then we are asked to consider multiple kinds of actors, both human and nonhuman alike. According to Latour, things, artifacts, and institutions may exert agency because they are part of this network of associations and affect its continuous reassemblage. In these networks, agency is not steered by human willpower (e.g., as an act of resistance) but by a variety of sources that "make a difference," as Latour says. Furthermore, an actor should not be seen as the origin of an action, but, according to Latour, "an actor is what is made *to act* by many others."[9] If "action is limited a priori to what 'intentional,' 'meaningful' humans do, it is hard to see how a hammer, a basket, a door closer, a cat, a rug, a mug, a list, or a tag could act." Yet if the social is considered an endless number of flexible associations, "then any thing that does modify a state of affairs by *making a difference* is an actor." The crucial question then is whether something "makes a difference in the course of some other agent's action or not." Fetching provisions with or without a basket, hitting a nail with or without a hammer, getting groceries with or without a list makes a difference, even though the list or the basket do not determine the action; rather, they "authorize, allow, afford, encourage, permit, suggest, influence, block, render possible, forbid, and so on."[10]

In the 1970s, Americans widely discussed whether running with or without Body Punch (or other energy drinks) made a difference, and what kind of diet made what kind of difference in the pursuit of fitness. As I argue in this chapter, in the early 1970s, runners, running manuals, and running magazines did not devote much thought to the effects of eating and drinking right on runners' lives and athletic performance, whereas by the end of the decade, these issues were very much in the spotlight and a subject of fervent debate. In the late 1970s, shaping up, taking good care of oneself, entering the kingdom of the well, and being a successful liberal citizen were widely perceived as being impossible without a proper diet. Let me underline at this point that I am neither seeking to prove how knowledge about the real effects of a proper diet on a runner's performance developed and spread in the 1970s nor am I trying to decipher the hype for energy drinks such as E.R.G., Body Punch, or Body Ammo as a fetish. Rather, I argue how eating right was charged with meaning and power in 1970s America and became what Latour calls a *factish*: fabricated knowledge that acquires shape as a "thing," which is a product and truth effect of discourses and cultural practices but which nevertheless really makes a difference.[11] Therefore, what makes a difference and what does not, or what is acknowledged as making a difference and therefore as being an actor, is embedded in history. To put it differently, the power of Body Punch and of the promises it makes to those who drink it is real, culturally charged, and deeply historical.

Some preliminary remarks on *Runner's World* and the meaning of running

As the story goes, in 1966, eighteen-year-old Bob Anderson from Manhattan, Kansas, was a dedicated runner looking for guidance on how to prepare for a marathon. Unable to find the information that he sought, Anderson went on to self-publish his own magazine, with two editions per year and a circulation of about five hundred copies. A few years later, Anderson sold 3,000 copies of six annual editions, brought another dedicated runner and journalist, Joe Henderson, onto the editorial team, and relocated the publication's headquarters to Mountain View, California, located in the Silicon Valley, the hub of the new high-tech economy and a burgeoning fitness and running Mecca. The magazine, henceforth called *Runner's World*, thrived with the running boom. While the number of Americans who considered themselves runners grew from two million in 1970 to thirty million in 1980, and the membership of the National Jogging Association multiplied exponentially,[12] the circulation of *Runner's World* grew from a few thousand copies and six editions per year in 1970 to a monthly publication of 500,000 copies by the end of the decade.[13]

First and foremost, *Runner's World* presented running as much more than a habit; it became a lifestyle dedicated to health and well-being, pleasure, and success. Since the early 1950s, a discourse made up of numerous voices had been pointing to the risks of American postwar life and the importance of taking up physical activity. A burgeoning consumer culture of yet unknown proportions helped ensure that Americans had televisions, automobiles, suburban houses, and unlimited amounts of food and drink. And after decades of economic depression, mobilization, and war, the sedentary, well-fed, and hard-drinking republic was increasingly seen as both a blessing and a curse. This lifestyle was praised as indicating the power and success of capitalism, yet it was also criticized for its degenerative effects. These sequelae of affluence were seen as a particular threat to middle-class American men in their forties, who were described as being exposed to many of the most serious risk factors: too much food and drink, not enough physical activity, high-stress jobs, and the onset of an age- and lifestyle-related clogging of the coronary arteries threatened to render them incapable of fulfilling their tasks as citizens of a liberal society, which was conceived as being founded upon the work of productive, energetic men.[14]

In the 1950s and 1960s, large male bodies were increasingly discussed by both the medical establishment and a larger public as unfit and potentially paralyzing for America, yet stout, mid-aged men still viewed themselves as quite normal.[15] In the ME society of the 1970s, however, unfitness became increasingly problematic for the self-image. It was at odds with male self-perceptions and also seen as a serious threat to American society at large. Running appeared to offer a welcome correction to the intemperate, sedentary lifestyle of postwar America, and as such, it had different connotations that might at first seem contradictory. On the one hand, the running craze was connected to a countercultural critique of the postwar ideal linking the good life with mass consumption, while on the other hand, sports and exercise themselves constituted a rapidly expanding consumer market in the 1970s and 1980s. Moreover, running was seen as a countercultural escape from the stresses of modern life, and yet to the extent that runners used it to exercise their capacity for self-improvement, they inadvertently became poster boys for a neoliberal culture that revolved around "ME" and its corporeal perfection. Their fit bodies became physical manifestations of health, ability, and efficiency in a society that was more market driven than ever.[16] *Runner's World* contributed to shaping all of these connotations. First, it nourished a self-perception of runners as belonging to a counterculture; second, it fostered running as a substantial part of the growing sports and exercise market; and third, it shaped runners as models of a productive life style, caring for their potential, their individual health, and the health of the nation.[17]

Running was described as having many meanings and purposes in addition to mere physical fitness. Runners ran for recreation, socialization, tranquility, sex appeal, or for medals and honors. But, as *Runner's World* stressed, no matter which purpose was being pursued, running never provided immediate gratification, "as fitness can't be stored. It must be earned over and over, indefinitely."[18] Therefore, taking up running meant more than merely adding another habit to one's daily routine. It meant changing one's whole lifestyle. Jogger Dave Mullens, who had just joined a group of early morning runners in Palo Alto, California, who called themselves the "Dawn Patrol," stressed with the fervor of an evangelical Christian that running "has really changed my entire existence around." Commentators and magazine articles repeated this message over and over again.[19]

White, middle-class men in their forties were most receptive to the idea of changing their lifestyle, which, according to historian Hillel Schwartz, appears to be a pattern that dates back to the nineteenth century.[20] In the 1970s, middle-aged and middle-class men were prompted to tend to their personal fitness by a daily avalanche of news stories, magazine articles, advice columns, and commercials. Steve Totten, founder of the Palo Alto running group "Dawn Patrol" and director of health and physical education at the regional branch of the Young Men's Christian Association (YMCA), pointed to the peer pressure that existed "especially among professional people, who are starting to realize the importance of fitness."[21] From early on, *Runner's World* stereotyped the generic jogger as "a man over 40 and desk chained all day ... who suddenly realizes his physical condition isn't what it should be."[22] As one reader complained to medical doctor and runner George Sheehan, a legend in running culture and author of a regular advice column in *Runner's World*, as soon as men reach "serious" middle age, "fat starts taking over ... then and only then do we lose control of our bodies."[23] This correlation between age, body shape, and self-control was supported by several public health surveys in the 1970s.[24] As studies of gender and race in modern history have convincingly argued, the performance of control over oneself and—maybe even more important—the cultural, social, and political recognition of this self-control have always been seen as evidence of one's ability and right to claim citizenship and participate in a society governed through freedom. Performances of this kind as well as the recognition of them have been highly gendered and racialized.[25] While the 1970s fat discourse surrounding women very much revolved around beauty and sexual attraction, for white, middle-class men, body fat and disease represented a loss of control and were seen as threatening to their hegemonic position in American society.[26] In the 1970s, this hegemony was more embattled than ever before due to the dual threats of black power and the women's movement, and thus, it was more important than ever for white men to regain control over their bodies. For 1970s men, being slim was less about beauty and attractiveness than about their productivity and fitness. Like a mantra, *Runner's World* repeated the phrase "jogging isn't enough."[27] To achieve the desired goals, it required more than taking up the habit of running, but also meant avoiding cigarettes and alcohol and eating right. In short, American men were asked to "live like a marathoner" so that they could exploit their potential and achieve "true fitness," meaning "less disease and a longer life!"[28]

From the early 1970s on, there was little doubt that eating right was critical for the fitness of runners. Yet it remained to be clarified what exactly "eating right" meant. A 1975 book titled *Food for Fitness* was promoted with a slogan that underscored the agency and power of food by stressing that "the difference a diet makes may be the difference between mediocrity and success."[29] By the mid-1970s, American runners became obsessed with eating right, and diet was poised to replace "intervals and speedwork as the prime topic of conversation among runners," as *Runner's World* stated at the end of the decade, when Americans were reportedly spending $500 million annually on their food faddism.[30] Doctor George Sheehan's medical advice column was full of questions from runners who wanted to know more about nutrition, and Americans were highly sensitive to the meaning of food as proper "fuel" for the body, a metaphor that had been around for almost a century but that was gaining historic momentum with the energy crises of 1973 and 1979.[31] Tables designed to express the relation between calorie intake, speed, and "mileage" were ubiquitous in the magazine,[32] and metaphors of the human motor "running on empty" and "the body's fuel tank" were most popular illustrations of the meaning of food for achieving peak performance.[33]

Food gained shape as a *factish* in American running culture in three different fields. First, runners wanted to know which diet was best for them in their everyday lives. Second, they wondered how and what to eat when preparing for a race. Third, they sought to find out what eating and, in this case, drinking right meant during a run and in particular during a race. Pursuing fitness had become a complicated matter, and it required learning more about "the difference a diet makes," as the *Food for Fitness* ad in *Runner's World* asserted.

Eating right in everyday life

Until the beginning of the 1970s, few runners were interested in questions pertaining to food. Yet early in the ME decade, readers began to urge *Runner's World* to say more about eating right, a topic editors confessed to having previously neglected. Fitness aficionados were obviously hoping that food would unlock a hidden source of strength and endurance. They got more of this help and advice when Sheehan, a dedicated runner, author, and cardiologist joined the magazine's editorial team.[34]

Early articles about the importance of nutrition in everyday life started popping up in 1971 and 1972. Their general idea was to draw the attention of more runners to the significance and power of food. These articles covered everything from body fat to nutrients, and from eating patterns to food intolerances, yet their basic message remained fairly simple: the "basic four"—milk, fruits and vegetables, meat, and grains—would give runners all they needed.[35]

In the following years, the topics of daily nutrition and fitness developed into a real "dietary faddism," as a lead article on "What Diet Can Do" pointed out—a title that explicitly resonated with the increasingly widespread belief in the agency of food to positively influence the performance of the runner.[36] Confused readers kept asking so many questions that Sheehan eventually grew tired of responding. After all, in the early 1970s he was not yet able to provide his readers with clear answers to many of their questions.[37] Here, the body-as-machine and fuel metaphors seemed helpful in making the power of food and eating right more tangible to runners and readers. A new magazine called *Fitness for Living* hyped itself as being an "owner's manual for your body."[38] At the end of the 1970s, eating right in the pursuit of fitness even became an existential question of Shakespearian proportion with the publication of an article entitled "To Eat Or Not to Eat."[39] Advice books were designed to guide runners through the complex field of diet and nutrition,[40] and special recipe collections promised to make "eating as much fun as running."[41]

Among the many topics pertaining to the power of food and eating in everyday life, two issues were debated with particular intensity: meat and food supplements. Early articles about dietary supplements were clearly opposed to the taking of extra doses of potassium, magnesium, and vitamins because putting foreign substances of any kind into one's body was frowned upon in "a drug-oriented society."[42] Yet this hesitation to pop pills quickly faded and was replaced by a belief in the power of food supplements. By stressing that "I am 43 years old and hope to break three hours in the marathon, and I wish it took only a vitamin pill," a reader expressed the desire of many runners who were eager to make their daily effort and dedication to fitness more efficient and also less strenuous.[43] Over the years, literature on food supplements acquired a particularly scientific aura, with expert voices providing complex explanations, including graphs, tables, and even footnotes, intended to underscore the arguments and lend them even greater persuasive power.[44] This information gave runners the feeling of possessing substantial knowledge on important medical issues. Toward the end of the decade, vitamins in particular were said to be crucial not as fuel for the body per se but rather as a way of assisting the body to more efficiently utilize fuel and oxygen. The promise that "by watching the foods you eat, [by] making certain to balance your intake of vitamins, you can live closer to your physical potential"[45] and keep on feeling "young and physically active through the course of [y]our lives"[46] seemed convincing to the ever-growing community of fitness aficionados. In the late 1970s, about half of all runners were reportedly taking nutritional supplements, which had acquired a reputation for making them better runners and thus healthier and better persons.[47] *Runner's World* equipped its readers with vitamin guides so that they would know exactly how the different vitamins were helping them in their pursuit of fitness and health.[48] Commercial products such as the "Champion Super Vitamin Mineral Formula" were marketed as making this endeavor easier by providing everything that was needed to improve a man's "natural ability to make a champion" in a single pill. They promised to runners that "*you can beat the energy crisis—and Champion makes the difference.*"[49]

The second big issue drawing attention in the everyday diet was the question of protein. In the early 1970s, Americans and most runners still believed protein to be a vital source of strength and therefore viewed eating meat as crucial in achieving peak fitness.[50] However, beginning with the counterculture of the late 1960s and early 1970s, and with the publication of Frances Moore Lappé's *Diet for a Small Planet*, vegetarianism began to take stronger root in American culture.[51] Vegetarian cookbooks, restaurants, and communes started to crop up around the country, especially in California. More than anything else, Lappé made an ecological argument against eating meat, a perspective many runners shared in principle and claimed for themselves and their lifestyle. Some people rejected meat for ecological reasons, while others rejected it on moral, spiritual, or health grounds. Others gave up meat to purge themselves of the toxic waste of modern society and keep the "body-temple" clean.[52]

Among runners, a slight skepticism toward eating meat was already noticeable by the early 1970s, when *Runner's World* advised its readers to skip meat immediately before hard runs and races because it was difficult to digest. Nevertheless, in 1973 the first extensive article on "What Diet Can Do" in *Runner's World* devoted a mere seven lines out of eight pages to vegetarianism, stating only briefly that the latest evidence suggested "that runners have no unusual need for protein."[53] Yet it took until the end of the decade for interest in vegetarianism to develop a broad base among runners, when running legend Amby Burfoot started to contribute articles to *Runner's World.* In 1968, Burfoot had been the last US winner of the Boston Marathon, which at that time was considered the most important race on the planet. Burfoot was nicknamed "the meatless runner," and he presented a passionate but careful argument for a vegetarian diet that would correct potential protein deficits.[54] A few months later, a follow-up article stressed that good running foods were those that were low in fat, high in carbohydrates, and that carried oxygen, meaning grain products, fruits, and vegetables, and not meat. "What the runner is craving, we know now, is not the steak, but the potato.... Glycogen is the primary muscle fuel, and like gas in your gas tank, the more you have in your muscles, the longer you can run.... If you want to run, you've got to have the proper fuel.... The runner who eats red meat, eggs and dairy products is putting oil in his gas tank."[55]

At the end of the decade, fitness aficionados had come a long way, from believing in protein as a source of strength to "knowing" that "in fact, excess protein can be detrimental to performance."[56] Meat had previously been associated with strength and energy, but by the late 1970s, runners had learned that digesting meat and the toxic wastes it left in their bodies cost them more energy than it provided. This transformation in knowledge was reiterated by late-1970s fitness iconography. *Runner's World* published a 1979 article on "Living without Meat" with a painted, two-page image of a bearded hippie runner sitting in the midst of salads and greens with a look in his eyes. And in June 1981, the new magazine *Fitness & Diet* displayed on its inaugural cover an image of a young woman with a seductive look biting into an apple.

Eating right before a race

Besides their daily diet, many runners considered the question of what to eat before a race as being of critical importance for improving their potential. In particular, carbohydrate loading was a big topic among runners. In the early 1970s, "carb loading" was still a mysterious practice that was shrouded in a fog of mixed information for most runners, making it difficult to come to an informed decision about whether or not to practice it as well as how to go about it if they did want to try it. The story of a runner who had "overloaded" and become sick by eating several loafs of bread in attempt to fill up his glycogen stores before a race stirred up confusion and an intense discussion for more than a year.[57] Nevertheless, in the mid-1970s the idea of improving performance through carbo loading was on those runners' minds who took a competitive approach to exercise. After all, it promised to help them shave precious minutes off of their times. The increasingly scientific presentation of this topic with graphs and tables provides clues about how seriously the search for a seemingly objective, practicable truth on this matter was taken.[58]

Toward the end of the decade, there was no doubt left that carb loading "made a difference" and offered a competitive advantage, at least when it came to long races. Everybody was said to do it, and, as *Runner's World* also noted, in the days before a race everybody turned vegetarian. The longer the race, the more important it was to overstock the "fuel tank" with carbs, and succeeding in a marathon was viewed as impossible without the right eating practice in the week before the race. By the late 1970s, it was established knowledge that sudden and radical changes in the diet were to be avoided, and runners who exaggerated their carb loading had become the object of ridicule. For a growing mass of runners, being aware of a few basic nutritional facts provided the key to sensible eating and successful running.[59]

Drinking right during a race

By and large, the knowledge on eating and fitness was presented in three different fashions. First, as emphasized earlier, its presentation was given a design that was intended to create a "scientific" aura. Medical doctors shared their truths about the best diet and the difference it could make by using charts, graphs, and tables, sometimes even including microscopic images, footnotes, and references to further readings. The second fountain of authority was the individual experience of other, typically more advanced runners. These were peers telling the "truth" about the effects certain kinds of food and drink had on their performance. The third type of knowledge presentation was the advice column, which was a mixture of both: fitness peers talked about their experiences and an expert (usually also a [male] runner) put them into context and responded with all of his knowledge.

In the early years, information about the intake of energy during a run was rare, and if available it came in the second type of presentation mentioned above, which was the anecdotal fashion. The first piece of this kind was published in March 1972, when runner Tom Sturak told the story of how he had come across a mysterious drink named E.R.G., sold in a totally unmarketable fashion. The acronym stood for "Electrolyte Replacement with Glucose," a drink made of water, lemonade, salt, and sugar. In the early

1970s, Gatorade had already been invented, but was predominantly focused on the football market, while E.R.G. was the only energy drink known on the running scene. It polarized runners. Some described the concoction as disgusting, while others considered it a sort of magical wonder drink that helped "replace what I lose when running." E.R.G. had been developed by a runner named Bill Gookin in self-experiments over many years, and as the myth went, it helped him finish the hilly Santa Barbara Marathon on a hot and dry day in under 2:30 hours at the age of 39 even after he had been feeling miserable at mid-race. "That made a believer out of me," Sturak later confessed.[60]

In the following years, E.R.G. regularly advertised in *Runner's World.* Often covering a whole page, the ads repeated Gookin's personal story of fitness, potential, improvement, and the success of a runner who beat his age and his weakness with the help of Gookinaid (as it was nicknamed after its creator) and "caught the young leaders ... coming up a long hill three miles from the finish." In language that highlighted the drink's agency and power, which was exactly what potential buyers expected, the ad stressed that "E.R.G. makes a difference in the way you run—so much of a difference, you'll have to try it to believe it."[61]

More and more runners followed this advice and tried E.R.G. The controversial debate over the problems associated with carbohydrate overloading further convinced them to be more moderate before the race and simply "take stuff on the road." Readers were a little insecure about when and how much to drink during a race and whether the "substance" they were taking does "really do the job." But in general, their comments praised E.R.G. as extremely powerful and helpful.[62]

In the second half of the 1970s, the market for energy drinks exploded. In contrast to E.R.G., manufacturers started to pick names that were meant to express the power contained in their foodstuffs and how they provided extra energy to the body. Products such as Body Punch or Body Ammo also promised to make a difference and power runners to "top performances." Their producers handed out free T-shirts so that runners could spread their gospel and demonstrate that they belonged to the growing community of runners who believed in the culture of the body, the pursuit of fitness, and the power of the product. A special belt and special bottle called "Drink on the Run" had also been designed, making it easier for fitness aficionados to take their drinks along on their routes.[63]

At the end of the decade, runners had a choice between many different types of energy drinks. They were embedded in an explosively growing running consumer culture that had expanded to include running shoes, clothes, and events. Just take the New York Marathon, for example, which grew from 126 starters in 1970 to more than 16,000 in 1980.[64] All the energy drinks on the market promised to facilitate effort, expand potential, and optimize performance by making the human motor run longer and faster. Runners loved this perspective. There was no doubt left that drinking right on the run was important, and all the energy drinks boasted in familiar wording that they made a difference. By the start of the 1980s, E.R.G. had lost its unique position on the market, but it nevertheless sought to point out that it was the original by stating in an advertisement in all-capital letters that "E.R.G. IS THE DIFFERENCE!"[65]

"The good, the bad, and the edible"

"The runner," writes historian Lynn Luciano in her study on male body images in modern America, "was the exemplary athlete for the Me Decade."[66] In their pursuit of a fit and firm body, runners were first and foremost competing with themselves in their efforts to fully explore their potential.[67] As historian Benjamin Rader argues, in the 1970s a new type of strenuous life was gaining shape, which was more than anything else aimed at the self.[68]

However, this self needed to be performed, for instance, by wearing one of the many T-shirts expressing the appreciation of the fit lifestyle and a willingness to work on one's health and potential. Therefore, as marathon legend Burfoot wrote in *Runner's World* at the dawn of the new decade, the fit body represented more than fitness. It stood for a general strenuousness, self-responsibility, stress management, environmental sensibility, and nutritional awareness.[69] Diet, runners had learned over the decade, "measurably affects performance in running and other sports," as *Runner's World* pointed out again and again.[70] The knowledge that food and eating right made a difference nudged the individual runner to act in a way deemed enhancing and productive.

Yet fitness as a norm and a practice was not bound to the field of sports and exercise. On the contrary, fitness was far more powerful, and, with a nod to Jonathan Metzl and Anna Kirkland,[71] "the new morality" of the neoliberal age. Exploring and using one's potential was the key quality of the ME society, and more than ever, eating right became a practice of good citizenship, as food scholar Charlotte Biltekoff has pointed out.[72] It was seen as proof of the ability to use one's freedoms properly and productively. The counterimage of the fit body was the fat body, seen as the physical embodiment of laziness, irresponsibility, a lack of environmental sensibility, and nutritional ignorance. The modern concept of the fat personality began to gain shape, one which succumbed to the temptations of America's extremely powerful sedentary lifestyle and food culture, providing, in the words of *Runner's World* nutrition author Virginia DeMoss "too many calories, too much fat, too much sugar and salt, and too little fiber, vitamins and other nutrients."[73] Thus the agency of foodstuffs and the power of eating right reached far beyond running and the runner, influencing—to recall Sontag's critique—who would obtain citizenship to the kingdom of the well and who would be ostracized to "that other place."[74]

Notes

1 Susan Sontag, *Illness as a Metaphor* (New York: Farrar, Straus and Giroux, 1978), 3; first published in *New York Review of Books*, January 26, 1978.

2 Pirkko Markula and Richard Pringle, *Foucault, Sport and Exercise: Power, Knowledge and Transforming the Self* (London: Routledge, 2006).

3 Tom Wolfe, "The 'Me' Decade and the Third Great Awakening," *New York Magazine*, August 23, 1976, accessed July 26, 2015, http://nymag.com/news/features/45938/.

4 Quoted after Charles Edgely, Betty Edgely, and Ronny Turner, "The Rhetoric of Aerobics: Physical Fitness as Religion," *Free Inquiry in Creative Sociology* 10, no. 2 (1982): 188.

5 Bill Ashcroft, Gareth Griffiths, and Helen Tifin, *Post-Colonial Studies: The Key Concepts* (London: Routledge, 2000), 6–7.

6 Alf Lüdtke, "Geschichte und Eigensinn," in *Alltagskultur, Subjektivität und Geschichte: Zur Theorie und Praxis von Alltagsgeschichte*, ed. Berliner Geschichtswerkstatt (Münster: Westfälisches Dampfboot Verlag, 1994), 139–53.

7 Nikolas Rose, *Powers of Freedom: Reframing Political Thought* (Cambridge: Cambridge University Press, 1999).

8 Sontag, *Illness as a Metaphor*, 3.

9 Bruno Latour, *Reassembling the Social: An Introduction to Actor-Network-Theory* (Oxford: Oxford University Press, 2005), 46.

10 Latour, *Reassembling the Social*, 2005, 59, 71–2 [italics mine].

11 Bruno Latour, *Pandora's Hope: Essays on the Reality of Science Studies* (Cambridge, MA: Harvard University Press, 1999), 266–92.

12 Gary Olsen, "National Jogging Association," *Runner's World* 8, no. 1 (January 1973): 35–7.

13 Jonathan Black, *Making the American Body* (Lincoln: University of Nebraska Press, 2013), 77; Shelly McKenzie, *Getting Physical: The Rise of Fitness Culture in America* (Lawrence: University Press of Kansas, 2013), 129.

14 William G. Rothstein, *Public Health and the Risk Factor: A History of an Uneven Medical Revolution* (Rochester, NY: University of Rochester Press, 2003); McKenzie, *Getting Physical*.

15 Sander L. Gilman, *Fat Boys: A Slim Book* (Lincoln: University of Nebraska Press, 2004), 5; Robert Kemp, *Nobody Need Be Fat* (London: William Heinemann, 1959), 33.

16 Darcy C. Plymire, "Positive Addiction: Running and Human Potential in the 1970s," *Journal of Sport History* 31, no. 3 (2004), 297–315.

17 Olsen, "National Jogging Association," 35–7.

18 Ted Corbitt, "Adjusting to Advancing Age," *Runner's World* 6, no. 6 (November 1971), 29.

19 Richard Hanner, "Beginning Running," *Runner's World* 14, no. 7 (July 1979), 68–71.

20 Hillel Schwartz, *Never Satisfied: A Cultural History of Diets, Fantasies, and Fat* (New York: The Free Press, 1986), 11; Gilman, *Fat Boys*, 4.

21 Hanner, "Beginning Running," 68–71.

22 John A. Kelley, "The Way to Start Running," *Runner's World* 9, no. 5 (May 1974), 19.

23 George Sheehan, Medical Advice, *Runner's World* 10, no. 3 (March 1975), 40.

24 Gilman, *Fat Boys*, 19.

25 Eric Foner, "The Meaning of Freedom in the Age of Emancipation," *Journal of American History* 81, no. 2 (1994), 435–60; Jürgen Martschukat and Olaf Stieglitz, *Geschichte der Männlichkeiten* (Frankfurt/M.: Campus, 2008).

26 Amy Erdman Farrell, *Fat Shame: Stigma and the Fat Body in American Culture* (New York: New York University Press, 2011).

27 Percy Cerutti, "Jogging Isn't Enough," *Runner's World* 6, no. 4 (July 1971), 36.

28 Thomas Bassler, "Live Like a Marathoner," *Runner's World* 9, no. 10 (October 1974), 26.

29 George Sheehan, Medical Advice, *Runner's World* 10, no. 3 (March 1975), 48; ads in *Runner's World* 10, no. 5 (May 1975); *Runner's World* 10, no. 6 (June 1975) and in many other issues.

30 Walter Rotkis, "A Simple Guide to Carbohydrate-Loading," *Runner's World* 14, no. 8 (August 1979), 30–1.

31 Carolyn T. de la Peña, *The Body Electric: How Strange Machines Built the Modern American* (New York: New York University Press, 2003).

32 For example, Alan Claremont, "Fuels for Extra Speed and Mileage," *Runner's World* 10, no. 6 (June 1975), 39; Norbert Sander, "Light at the End of the Run: A Good Running Program Can Be the Best Weight Control," *Runner's World* 14, no. 5 (May 1979), 96–103.

33 For example, "The Valuable Art of Fasting," *Runner's World* 13, no. 6 (June 1978), 61–3; Jim Lekiem, "The Role of the B Vitamins in Daily Life: If the Body's Fuel Tank Comes Up Short on Vitamin B the Long Run Could Come Up Short," *Runner's World* 14, no. 9 (September 1979), 59–61.

34 Black, *Making the American Body*, 76–7.

35 "What's New in Nutrition," *Runner's World* 6, no. 6 (November 1971), 36; Ralph Bircher, Tom Sturak, and George Sheehan, "Eat, Drink, and Be Weary," *Runner's World* 7, no. 2 (March 1972), 32–5.

36 "What Diet Can Do: New Evidence on What Eating and Drinking Mean to Times and Distances," *Runner's World* 10, no. 7 (July 1973), 8–15.

37 George Sheehan, "Medical Advice," *Runner's World* 9, no. 6 (June 1974), 42.

38 Advertisement for *Fitness for Living* in *Runner's World* 10, no. 9 (September 1973), 15

39 David Higdon, "To Eat Or Not to Eat," *Runner's World* 13, no. 1 (January 1978), 44–8.

40 Runner's World, *Food for Fitness* (Mountain View, CA: World Publications, 1975) and Runner's World, *The Complete Diet Guide for Runners and Other Athletes* (Mountain View, CA: World Publications, 1978).

41 Joanne Milkereit and Hal Higdon, *Runner's Cookbook* (Mountain View, CA: World Publication, 1979); Nathan Pritikin, *The Pritikin Program for Diet and Exercise* (New York: Bantam, 1979); Joanne Milkereit and Hal Higdon, "Eating Right to Run Right: Recipes That Can Make Eating as Much Fun as Running," *Runner's World* 14, no. 5 (May 1979), 58–65.

42 Gabe Mirkin, "Super Foods?" *Runner's World* 7, no. 6 (November 1972), 25.

43 "What Diet Can Do," 8–15.

44 Claremont, "Fuels for Extra Speed and Mileage," 39.

45 Lekiem, "The Role of the B Vitamins in Daily Life," 59–61.

46 Michael Weiner and Jonathan Rothschild, "The Vitamin That Likes Oxygen: A Runner Can Increase the Use of Oxygen by Carefully Using Vitamin E," *Runner's World* 15, no. 2 (February 1980), 87–9.

47 Higdon, "To Eat Or Not to Eat," 44–8.

48 Viginia DeMoss, "The Complete Vitamin Guide: Everything the Runner Needs to Know about the Wonderful World of Vitamins," *Runner's World* 15, no. 4 (April 1980), 34–9.

49 Advertisements for Champion Super Vitamin Mineral Formula, *Runner's World* 14, no. 9 (September 1979), 110, and *Runner's World* 15, no. 1 (January 1980), italics in the original.

50 Gilman, *Fat Boys*, 194.

51 Frances Moore Lappé, *Diet for a Small Planet* (New York: Ballantine Books, 1971).

52 Warren Belasco, *Appetite for Change: How the Counterculture Took On the Food Industry*, 2nd ed. (Ithaca, NY: Cornell University Press, 2006), 56–61; Harvey Levenstein, *Paradox of Plenty: A Social History of Eating in Modern America*, 2nd ed. (Berkeley: University of California Press, 2003), 178–85.

53 "What Diet Can Do," 8–15.

54 Amby Burfoot, "The Meatless Runner," *Runner's World* 13, no. 2 (February 1978), 48–55.

55 Julian Whitaker, "Diet Shortcuts to Oxygen Uptake: A Runner Can Sometimes Work His Best Training Miracles at the Dining-Room Table," *Runner's World* 13, no. 5 (May 1978), 72–3.

56 Julian Whitaker, "How Much Protein Do Runners Need?" *Runner's World* 14, no. 2 (February 1979), 66–7

57 "What's New in Nutrition," *Runner's World* 6, no. 6 (June 1971), 36–9; George Sheehan, Medical Advice, *Runner's World* 10, no. 3 (1975), 40; "What Diet Can Do," 8–15.

58 "Solid and Liquid Energy," *Runner's World* 9, no. 7 (July 1974), 29–31; "Bob Fitts: The Modified Diet Act," *Runner's World* 9, no. 10 (October 1974), 37; Paul Slovic, "Eating Away Precious Minutes," *Runner's World* 10, no. 11 (November 1974), 34–5.

59 "The Marathon: 10 Steps to Improvement," *Runner's World* 13, no. 2 (February 1978), 83; Roy Bruder, "Nature's Carbo-Loading Secrets," *Runner's World* 13, no. 4 (Apr. 1978), 50–1; Amby Burfoot, "The Joys of Vegetarian Carbohydrate-Loading," *Runner's World* 14, no. 1 (Jan. 1979), 138; Rotkis, "A Simple Guide," 30–1; Steven Subotnick, "9 Ways to Survive Marathons," *Runner's World* 15, no. 3 (March 1980), 82–3.

60 Bircher, Sturak, and Sheehan, "Eat, Drink, and Be Weary," 32–3.

61 Advertisement for E.R.G., *Runner's World* 8, no. 5 (May 1973), 41, and in *Runner's World* 10, no. 7 (July 1973), 44, and in *Runner's World* 10, no. 6 (June 1975).

62 Readers' Comments, *Runner's World* 9, no. 4 (April 1974), 47 and 9, no. 10 (October 1974), 40; "Solid and Liquid Energy," *Runner's World* 9, no. 7 (July 1974), 29–31.

63 Advertisement for Body Punch, *Runner's World* 12, no. 8 (August 1977), and 12, no. 9 (September 1977), and 13, no. 1 (January 1978); advertisement for Body Ammo, *Runner's World* 12, no. 12 (December 1977); advertisement for Drink on the Run, *Runner's World* 14, no. 7 (July 1979), 113.

64 McKenzie, *Getting Physical*, 131–2; Lynne Luciano, *Looking Good: Male Body Image in Modern America* (New York: Hill & Wang, 2001), 117.

65 Advertisment for E.R.G., *Runner's World* 13, no. 7 (July 1978), 105.

66 Luciano, *Looking Good*, 121

67 Plymire, "Positive Addiction," 297–315.

68 Benjamin G. Rader, "The Quest for Self-Sufficiency and the New Strenuosity: Reflections on the Strenuous Life of the 1970s and the 1980s," *Journal of Sport History* 18, no. 2 (1991), 255–66.

69 Amby Burfoot, "Eliminating the Need to Be Sick," *Runner's World* 15, no. 2 (February 1980), 79–81.

70 Advertisement for *Complete Diet Guide for Runners and Other Athletes*, *Runner's World* 13, no. 1 (January 1978), 76.

71 Jonathan Metzl and Anna Kirkland (eds.), *Against Health: How Health Became the New Morality* (New York: New York University Press, 2010).

72 Charlotte Biltekoff, *Eating Right in America: The Cultural Politics of Food and Health* (Durham, NC: Duke University Press, 2013), 93 and 98.

73 Virginia DeMoss, "The Good, the Bad & the Edible," *Runner's World* 15, no. 6 (June 1980), 39–45.

74 Sontag, *Illness as Metaphor*.

7

Being too big—as deviance from the societal order

Eva Barlösius

Food and power are closely interlinked in a complex web. Food is a result of power relations and is used to underscore and establish them. Virtually the entire spectrum of power inequalities is reflected in how food is allocated, which diets are valued or which are praised, and how food-related precepts and regulations come to be adopted. Whether it is a question of power relations between the governing and the governed, insiders and outsiders, or majorities and minorities, inequalities of power nearly always become apparent in the distribution, promotion, and denigration of foods and in dietary rules and duties. Food possesses this socially informative value regardless of whether the inequalities of power are due to political, social, cultural, or gender-specific forces.[1]

Ways of exerting of power

Outright food deprivation is surely the most violent way of using food to wield power. However, providing food in a physiologically *un*objectionable manner is also an act of exerting power if culturally and socially inferior food is given, as the cultural anthropologist Margaret Mead illustrated with the example of postwar food distribution.[2] To win over the population of a defeated country, the victor distributes food that is culturally and socially valued in the occupied territory. Otherwise, the population would experience the distributed food as an additional humiliation.

Another way of brandishing power through food consists in promoting or denigrating styles of eating and cooking and in resorting to such judgments to produce and justify social favoritism or discrimination. Various eating styles and cuisines do not just serve as an expression and result of cultural diversity but also form part of a culinary hierarchy closely corresponding to the sociostructural hierarchy.[3] Examples are the differentiation between middle-class and proletarian cooking or between prestigious national cuisines and those associated with immigrant groups and other outsiders. Pierre Bourdieu's study *Distinction: A Social Critique of the Judgement of Taste* showed that taste thereby becomes the declared generator of cultural and social difference.[4] This social utilization of taste gives rise to cultural promotion and denigration of eating styles and cuisines—the specific processes of judgment that mesh with sociostructural disparities. The power of taste thus consists in highlighting differences and in creating and justifying inequalities.

Yet another mode of exercising power centers not on taste but rather on notions of "good" or "bad." It lays down the dietary rules and regulations to be heeded and, if violated, the punishments to be expected and upheld as legitimate. The use of power in declaring something good or bad consists in rewarding agreement with and sanctioning "deviance" from a given, socially binding "order of eating." The order of eating consists of rules of eating that are commonly recognized as obligatory. The use of food as an instrument of power becomes especially conspicuous in the way food-related moral prescriptions—eating ethics—are validated and imbued with their socially binding character. The fundamental dictates of eating ethics, such as sharing food, extend far beyond the order of eating. They simultaneously, sometimes even primarily, address key aspects of the social order. Moral precepts about fair distribution of food often correspond to societal agreement on social justice. It is no coincidence that major aspects of eating ethics accord with what is expected of the social order. After all, the order of eating is deemed the quintessential model of culture, and the consensus, as Gerhard Baudy suggests, is that "the social fabric emerged together with the distribution of food."[5] "Rules of eating are social rules par excellence," he explains. They greatly contribute to the drive "to maintain a social order itself."[6]

This chapter deals with this third way of bringing power to bear, that of imbuing a particular order of eating with social authority. I am especially interested in how the rules of eating spill over into the social order and, conversely, how rules of the social order are articulated and asserted through the order that governs eating. If these rules are grounded in knowledge, the distinction between good and bad is usually replaced by that between "right" and "wrong."[7] In contemporary societies—by which I mean nearly all late-industrial societies, especially those in Europe and North America—scientific knowledge has an almost complete monopoly on legitimacy. In these societies, a diet is acknowledged as being good if it is based on expertise in the health or nutritional sciences.[8] That kind of diet is considered right.

This way of exerting power can be studied with a number of examples: vegetarianism or veganism, ecological or biological diets, and meals wholly free of processed foods such as convenience or ready-to-eat products. However, these examples would concentrate the analysis on the question of how certain social groups aim to have a new order of eating win out and how they ensure its social acceptance. The best way to explore the interaction between the order of eating and the social order, as is true in general for examining social rules and the successful imposition of social order, is to investigate deviances and sanctions.[9] The potential for exercising power in those cases is greatest when social rules and social order have actually been or are presumed to have been violated and ignored.

In contemporary societies, "being too big" is one of the phenomena viewed as resulting from a "wrong" diet and, hence, from neglecting the order of eating.[10] The condition is also associated closely with social deviance from core values of the social order, such as self-discipline and a focus on achievement. Socially, politically, publicly, and scientifically, there is presumably no comparable phenomenon that draws the attention and the criticism that being too big does.[11] This physical condition is seen and often impugned as an alleged breach of and disrespect for the "right" ("healthy") diet and social rules, such as practicing self-control and showing initiative and commitment. A big body is thereby interpreted as an objectivation of deviance.[12]

Both the current view on being too big and society's interaction with people regarded as too big are rooted in a long history of how bodies, self-discipline, fitness, eating, and movement are interrelated. This history harkens back to the ancient world.[13] The modern outlook on the subject has been shaped especially by late nineteenth-century efforts to reform a person's way of life. At that time, bodies, self-discipline, fitness, food, and exercise were linked with each other in a way that survives to the present. The body still represents self-discipline and fitness, conditioning that requires nutritious food and exercise.[14] Whereas nineteenth-century reforms in a person's way of life were addressed primarily to the middle class, physical norms for the body have since become a standard for society as a whole.[15] They permeate the social order, particularly those strata whose societal integration is thought to be at risk.

Why the concept of stigmatization is insufficient

Much of the vast research on how society treats persons regarded as too big identifies their social experiences chiefly as stigmatization.[16] These studies document that big people are reproached for rejecting accepted norms and values, not sharing collective moral convictions, and failing to meet social expectations such as self-discipline and self-determination.[17] Stigmatization is particularly frequent on the job, in some media formats, and, in certain situations, in the health services. It is less common and less intense at school and in training programs.[18] Nonetheless, children as young as six or seven years associate obesity with negative character traits, including some that have nothing to do with weight.[19] Even three-year-olds tell stories that deprecate chubby and fat children, describing them as lazy, unattractive, unhappy, unloved, unfriendly, and sloppy.[20] They know and already use society's status-enhancing and status-degrading words to describe their own bodies and the bodies of others.[21] Children, thus, already experience (and reproduce) clear stigmatization at an early age.

Such analyses of stigmatization processes are indisputably important because they point out essential facets of society's response to obesity and to people regarded as overweight. As I contend below, however, they do not suffice to capture the full range of the ways in which people exert power by enforcing an order of eating and a social order tightly intertwined with it. The concept of stigmatization centers on the humiliation visited on people who are considered fat and on how they react to it. Reactions, activities, and actions that do not seem to have any direct connection with stigmatization go largely unstudied.

The reason for this omission rests on preconceived notions of where stigmatizations occurs and what it is about them that is socially significant. On the one hand, perspectives of this sort lead one to underestimate much of what it is like to be big. On the other hand, persons whom society treats as being too big are observed by sociological studies to find out what stigmatizations they have to face. This approach promotes a rather one-dimensional viewpoint and encourages the examination of processes to which social significance is imputed. To a person feeling excessively big by society's standards, the constant rebukes from the engineered physical environment may be highly salient because their documentation of the phenomenon's pervasiveness is especially unrelenting. By contrast, the explicit put-downs in school and training programs may tend to have a one-off character for these people. In most cases, however, the concept of stigmatization encompasses only the express form of the phenomenon.

Humiliation and disapproval can occur consciously or unconsciously. These attitudes are often expressed without any action or comment. This type of reprobation is especially common in the way the physical world is arranged, as with the width of seats or cubicles.[22] It gives rise to the unremitting reminder of being too big. The social message that one is too big is constantly experienced no matter what the observed persons do or where they are. They also sense this ubiquity even when it is not there in the minds of people who are thin. With the concept of stigmatization, however, society's way of dealing with obesity tends to be thought of only as reactions, activities, and actions that have a perceptible, visible, definite quality as far as people who are treated "normally" are concerned. More pointedly, these persons reconstruct the distinction between "fat" and "thin" from the perspective of being thin, that is, in terms of what society sees as normal. From this angle obesity represents deviance. To appropriately ascertain the social dynamics entailed—the social construction of the difference between "normal" and "deviant"—one must refer back to the social order as a key concept.[23] That link makes it possible to reconstruct the entire scope of what it means to exert power. In particular, it helps one understand why comparatively big people may react defensively even in situations that involve no censure for failing to conform to the order of eating and the social order.

Social order and its legitimation: A theoretical framework

To formulate a viable framework, I draw on Peter L. Berger and Thomas Luckmann's theory of the social construction of reality.[24] According to these researchers, the social order acquires its authority directly from the everyday world through a distinction between the "unproblematic" and the "problematic," that is, between what is normal and what deviates from the normal. Berger and Luckmann hold that social reality comes across to the individual as an "objective reality" and is thereby apt to give the false impression that the perceived characterization of social reality is based on fact. Berger and Luckmann, however, do not take the concept to mean that at all. "Objective" character is inherent in social reality because it comes across to people as institutional order and is experienced by them as a compelling fact emanating from outside. To illustrate this view, Berger and Luckmann say that objective reality consists of "objectivations" possessing two properties. First, they are "common goods" that are familiar to all members of a society on principle. Second, these objectivations are socially binding to a high degree. These two properties turn objectivations into institutions, which is why Berger and Luckmann usually speak of the totality of the institutional order rather than of objective reality.

Only when the institutional order has become a common good and is regarded as obligatory, write Berger and Luckmann, "does it become possible to speak of a social world at all, in the sense of a comprehensive and given reality confronting the individual in a manner analogous to the reality of the natural world."[25] At that point in the individual's mind, it possesses its "own reality" that needs legitimation.[26] In other words, the institutional world requires explanation and justification.[27] Legitimation imbues the institutional order with a "new meaning."[28] The existing social reality is justified. and it explains why that reality is as it is and not otherwise. The processes of legitimation extend to all of social reality, permitting "the totality of the institutional order" to "make sense."[29] Through legitimations "the 'first-order' objectivations that have been institutionalized" become "objectively available and subjectively plausible"[30] to the individual—that is, that they are known to that person and that he or she expressly agrees with them. Precisely that outcome is a social function of legitimation.[31]

Those people whose thinking or actions document that legitimations are not objectively available, subjectively plausible, or both, are treated like "actual or potential deviators" who threaten to veer from the "official definition of reality."[32] As Berger and Luckmann contend, society meets them with therapy so as to align them more closely to the social order. Therapies, they write, are rooted in "knowledge that includes a theory of deviance, a diagnostic apparatus, and conceptual system for the 'cure of souls'."[33] Therapies respond to the failure to heed legitimations and, like them, rest on bodies of knowledge permeated by values.

In the following pages, persons who are considered too big and who are treated accordingly by society are asked what position they have on dominant legitimations. The focus is partly on the order of eating and partly on those social legitimations according to which a "too big body" is seen as objectified deviance. More specifically, the present chapter asks, does deviance from the order of eating and the social order become objectified in a "too big body"?

The study thus encompasses two steps. First, I check whether knowledge about the "right diet" is objectively available to people who experience themselves as too big in society and whether, given this knowledge, they portray themselves in a subjectively plausible manner. Second, I inquire as to whether the purposefulness of the established legitimations is objectively available and subjectively plausible to these persons or whether they identify themselves as deviators.

The research project: Relatively big youth

The empirical foundation of this investigation was a major project on obesity among young people.[34] The subjects were young people because active and fundamental engagement with the everyday world is typical among members of this age group. They are especially keen on the difference between problematic and unproblematic. In addition, they customarily confront prevailing social legitimations intensely and are likely to take a clear stance on them. Most of the young people who participated in the study were attending either lower secondary school or a school for children with learning disabilities and difficulties. They found themselves in the phase of their lives in which they were aware that they would soon be held responsible for their social recognition and the part they play in society. This circumstance makes it especially interesting to learn how they position themselves in relation to dominant legitimations.

Data collection proceeded in three ways in this research project: (a) group discussions with relatively big young people from socially disadvantaged quarters of the city, (b) group discussions with parents of overweight children, and (c) a World Café with experts on practices for preventing overweight.[35] In this presentation I draw only on the group discussions with the young people, the complete transcripts of which are available.[36] Group discussion was selected as a method because it is particularly well suited to documenting collective patterns of orientation and experience, such as legitimations.[37] Thematically, the group discussions began with prompts stemming from Berger and Luckmann's notion of "society as objective reality," such as common typifications and objectivations of the everyday world and their social legitimation.[38] The later prompts inquired into subjective comments on the legitimations and explored expectations the participants had of their future biographical trajectory.

Eight group discussions were conducted with sixty boys and girls taking part. Each group consisted of six to ten persons, and the discussions lasted from an hour and a half to two hours. The discussions were segmented by gender, ancestry (German or Turkish), and age (11- to 13-year-olds and 14- to 16-year-olds). The young people had been recruited primarily from city quarters in which social reporting had recorded (a) an above-average percentage of the population to be receiving unemployment benefits or social welfare, (b) overrepresentation of persons with migration background in comparison to other city quarters with high quotas of dwellings under municipal occupancy regulations, and (c) other indices whose scores of sociospatial disadvantage were high. This sociospatial recruitment was intended to ensure that young people from socially disadvantaged families participated in the group discussions. The project concentrated on young people from the so called "underclass" because these children are mostly affected by being heavy.[39] Recruitment in the city quarters proceeded by means of fliers distributed in schools; in institutions promoting cultural activities, youth work, and health; and among pediatricians.[40]

The flier's title—the wordplay "Dicke Freunde?", meaning both "close friends" and "big friends"—proved highly effective, though it did not specify weight or girth. In keeping with the project's hypothesis that obesity was above all a social experience, the fliers were aimed at young people who perceived of themselves as too big. No medical criteria were set, though medically, most of the young people who attended the group discussions would be classifiable as overweight and obese. Only a few were grossly obese. The same approach was taken to categorizing the participants as German or Turkish.[41] The young people assigned themselves to one group or the other, with some of the parents doing so for them when registering their children for the study. For example, there were second- and third-generation children of Turkish migrants who signed into the "German group discussions" and others who attended the "Turkish rounds of discussion."

In the following pages, I analyze the portions of the group discussions that were intended to elicit the young people's comments on legitimations of the social order and of eating. Those pertaining to eating were not differentiated by gender, family background, or age, so the dissimilar compositions of the group discussions are not discussed further.[42]

Big rock candy mountain: An "inverse" world

When individuals or groups interacting with their social environment repeatedly receive the direct or indirect message that they deviate from recognized legitimations, it is not trivial matter to elicit their positions on themselves. Any attempt to broach the subject head-on is colored by normative expectations and social desires. To get a discussion going, I chose a narrative that describes an inverse world and builds on legitimations contrary to those that apply in the everyday world of the participants. This inversion was intended to enable the comparatively big young people to disassociate themselves from accepted legitimations without immediately laying themselves open to criticism as deviators.

The methodological considerations centered on Alfred Schütz and Thomas Luckmann's analysis of the fantasy world.[43] Contrasting the fantasy world and the life world is precisely what makes these both worlds appear closely interrelated. Fairy tales, according to these two authors, convey closed structures of meaning and therefore have their own web of legitimations. When talking about fantasy worlds—indeed, when fantasizing at all—people begin to distinguish between what is real and what is fictional. They separate the two. Engaging the participants with fantasy worlds thus started with a conversation about "objective social reality" and what characterizes it. "The knowledge we call upon," Schütz and Luckmann write, "to say what was and was not 'in reality', what exists 'only' in the dream, and what is the 'wrong' place and the 'wrong' time—that knowledge has its home in the natural attitude of daily life."[44] Contrasting fantasy world is well suited to encouraging people to talk about the "objective social reality." So we looked for fairy tales in which those legitimations are inversely presented, of which big people are said not only to disrespect them but also to deviate from them. We choose the traditional German version of the *Big Rock Candy Mountain*, the *Schlaraffenland*, in order to encourage the big young people to talk about legitimations of objective social reality, hoping that they would not directly refer to social expectations but how they might cope with societal legitimations.

The *Schlaraffenland* was an age-old fairy tale that about a "popular utopia," an imaginary place of ease and plenty.[45] The story of this fantasyland is widely known in Europe.[46] In the Netherlands it goes by the name *Luikkerland*; in England, *Lubberland* or *Cockaigne*; in Italy, *Cuccagna*; in Spain, *Cucaña*, in Germany, *Schlaraffenland* (the form of the story used in this study's group discussions); and in France, *Pays de Cocagne*. The oldest known surviving written text to mention the tale of this mythical place comes from France in the mid-thirteenth century. From the thirteenth through the nineteenth century, it was told and retold anew in most European countries.[47] In the nineteenth century, the Brothers Grimm edited it for children and included it in their collection entitled *Children's and Household Tales*.[48] The long history, wide circulation, numerous written versions, and linguistic reworking of the story, including the familiar US song "Big Rock Candy Mountain," indicate that it is "a fantasy transcending all periods."[49] It tells of ancient wishes and dreams, content that makes it understandable by persons unfamiliar with the story itself, for something resonating in it has the character of "common heritage."[50]

The special thing about this fairy tale is the way it depicts shared wishes and dreams. Literary criticism and the humanities identify the land of milk and honey as an inverse world because it praises the opposite of what is considered worthwhile and legitimate in the "real world."[51] The "inversion of prevailing norms," writes Werner Wunderlich, "runs through nearly all texts about a land of milk and honey."[52] It is a world in which idlers, slackers, and dalliers are welcome. Indeed, people *are supposed to be* lazy there. Whoever is nevertheless industrious and shows a zeal to work risks being whipped and expelled from this dream world. The social hierarchy is turned upside down. The less a person works and the dimmer he or she is, the higher he or she climbs on the social ladder. The dumbest and laziest person of all is chosen as the king.[53]

In most interpretations this fantasy land is an antithesis, or a counterpart (*Gegen-Bild*), of the "developing bourgeois world of modern times," especially its work ideology.[54] Other bourgeois virtues, too, such as moderation, reason, and goal directedness, are lampooned in the depiction. These interpretations give rise to another reason for using this tale as a prompt for group discussions: it caricatures those behaviors and legitimations that are regarded as obligatory in modern society as well and for which big people are reproached for ignoring. Big people are thus often described as lazy, immoderate, and listless underachievers unconcerned about the future (see part 2). On Big Rock Candy Mountain, however, these traits are not only esteemed but also are the only legitimate ones. The place is a self-contained sensory world of its own, a web of legitimations.

The idea behind presenting a world of converse meanings was to help the young people take a stance on its legitimations without immediately having to comment on justifications and explanations of the "real" order of eating and social order. In the group discussions, the participants worked out a children's abridged version of the German equivalent of Big Rock Candy Mountain—*Schlaraffenland*—by replacing archaic words with more recent ones to adapt the text to the language of the young people. But the fairy-tale character was retained to make it clear to them that the story was about a fantasy world.

Most of the young people had no awareness of the fairy tale. A few had a very rough idea of it. Despite this lack of familiarity, they associated the expression *Schlaraffenland* with a dream and fantasy world. Many of the participants began the discussion by calling the place fictional. They imagined what it would mean if this dream and fantasy world were real. Examples of their answers are as follows:

> If it is the way it's described there? (BT 14–16)[55]
> If it were actually there for real and ... (GD 11–13)
> But if that were really there. (GD 14–16)

As intended, the prompt moved the young people to compare the tale's conceived social reality with "real reality," to relate the meaningfulness of the one kind of legitimation to that of the other kind, and to explain their personal agreement and rejection in each case.

The proverbial land where milk and honey flow

The first part of the tale of *Schlaraffenland* conjures a place that is overflowing with the most desired foods and where gluttony is welcome. This description is intended to bring the young people to talk openly about their preferences—quite apart from the dominant order of eating. Not only is food overabundant in this land but also no attention is paid to things that are "right" or "wrong," "healthy" or "unhealthy." The order of eating in this land is based on whim and the pleasure of indulging oneself. This craving is all that counts as legitimate. It completely inverts contemporary society's order.

The prompt in the group discussion consisted of the passage describing the *Schlaraffenland* as a remote, mysterious place with a superabundance of the most wondrous foods, a land with "houses of gingerbread," "roofs of pancakes," and "garden fences of warm sausages." The "brooks flow with milk," and "fresh bread rolls grow" on trees. The prompt ends with the sentence "What a pity that no one knows the way to *Schlaraffenland*." The passage was projected onto the wall so that the young people could read along. They were asked afterward "to imagine you were in *Schlaraffenland*, where everything is possible and allowed, and everything you wish to have would appear on the table as if by magic. What would there be for you to eat and drink?"

Basically, two identifiable patterns emerged from their responses, which differed almost solely in the way they began. Typical of the first pattern was that the young people immediately named only foods and beverages that they were sure represented a diet recognized as right and good.

A: Maybe also some fresh fruit—watermelon, kiwis,
F: Apples, water, bananas,
C: Salads,
J: Fresh juices, too,
E: That's healthy. (GD 11–13)

This discussion sequence was an exchange between girls, but the same response pattern occurred in the boys' group discussion: "Well, if that really existed, then you'd also have to think about your health. If you were to wolf down McDonald's cheeseburgers every day here, you'd get sick. You could also wish for vegetables" (BD 11–13).

In the second response pattern, the young people spontaneously counted up what they wanted to eat in this land. After these rather casual statements, they began to qualify what they had just wished for by adding words like "maybe," "only a little," or "very rarely." The following discussion sequence exemplifies a transition from an initially unself-conscious listing to hedging:

F: Chicken,
K: A lot of milk,
A: Cheesecake,
C: Bread rolls,
A: Maybe cola. (GT 11–13)

The young people frequently hedged in this manner during the group discussions, immediately "correcting" their statements nearly every time they mentioned a food or beverage they liked if it was labeled as something wrong or unhealthy under the dominant order of eating. It was their way of accentuating their agreement with accepted dietary knowledge.

Throughout the group discussions, the young people strove to avoid reprobation and to stress the notions of what a right and good diet is when speaking about food. They were thus keenly aware of the legitimate knowledge that was considered right, and they repeated it as quickly and easily as they could say their simple multiplication tables. They were intent on showing that they understood the difference between healthy and unhealthy and right and wrong foods and beverages. But to these young people, there was more to it than just reciting knowledge of nutrition. They wanted to emphasize that the valuations woven into this knowledge were objectively available and subjectively plausible to them. Their verbalizations were aimed at affirming legitimations, not at reporting their own daily eating habits. The young people proffered their agreement with the accepted legitimations and their conformity to what is perceived as the official definition of reality. This response demonstrates the power that lies in legitimations and the threat of being labeled as "actual or potential deviators." The young people felt pressed to describe themselves in ways suggesting that their diets conformed to the established order of eating.

> I like eating a lot of fruit, though you can't tell from the way I look. (GT 14–16)
>
> I now eat one of those for supper, ... without anything on it and not fried in fat, either. (BD 11–13)

If, by mistake, the young people started a sentence in a way that might raise doubt about their views, they corrected themselves immediately and ended their comments with the moral distinction between good and bad:

> But the dumb thing is ... many unhealthy foods ... taste really good, but there are also enough healthy things that taste good. (GD 11–13)
>
> I'd bring something [to *Schlaraffenland*] that would only taste like McDonald's but have nothing in it like calories or anything like that. (BD 14–16)

Overall, the young people went to great lengths to correct themselves along the lines of the order of eating. It is thus quite unjustified to make the blanket assumption that relatively big young people have little or no knowledge about diet. They also grasped that it is about a kind of knowledge associated with showing respect, knowledge with which a person communicates his or her social conformity. They had internalized this message and constantly took care to monitor what they said about themselves. This behavior is precisely what documents the power of social rules and regulations based on a specified order of eating. The young people may not have been appropriately aware of the extent of that dominance until they realized that everyday reality presumably looks quite different. These two response patterns also surfaced in a preliminary study with relatively big children and young people and their counterparts who are thin. The two groups did not differ in their knowledge about a wholesome diet and exercise, but diverged markedly when speaking about what they liked to eat. Whereas the thinner children and young people spontaneously listed what they liked, the big children and young people first named foods considered healthy or corrected themselves as described above (see Barlösius and Philipps, 2015). Constant self-monitoring and self-correction when responding about the order of eating thus represented a typical behavioral pattern among relatively big children and young people.

The “inverse” for the “real” world

The second part of the story of the *Schlaraffenland* imparts a lesser-known alternative design: that of the working world, social recognition, and the hierarchy of inequality. This description of the land inverts three paramount legitimations of the social order: meritocratic orientation, sociostructural relegation, and social recognition and participation in society.

A. It is forbidden to work in the *Schlaraffenland*. Laziness is rewarded. This dictate contradicts the explanations and justifications of meritocratic society. It also indirectly addresses the way society deals with obesity because relatively big people are assumed to lack initiative (see above).

B. The laziest person occupies the highest social position. This arrangement, too, inverts accepted legitimations of the real world, in which social positions are assigned largely according to the meritocratic triad of education, occupation, and income. Big people often have the impression of being shunted into inferior and less respected positions because of their bodies.[56]

C. Diligent people have to leave the community inhabiting the *Schlaraffenland*. They are excluded. In the real world, participation in society comes mostly through paid work and active contributions. Once again, the fairy tale reverses the dominant legitimations. With comparatively big young people afraid of losing their social affiliation and ardently feeling the desire to belong, the third distinctive feature of the *Schlaraffenland*, too, ties into their personal experience.[57]

The prompt in the group discussions was, "What do people do in the *Schlaraffenland*? Whatever it is, they are not allowed to work, and the one who sleeps the latest is rewarded for it. The laziest person becomes king, and anyone who works too hard must leave the land." Although nothing about obesity or anything about big people was mentioned in this section or anywhere else in the tale, the young people immediately associated "not working," "sleeping in," and "the laziest person" with being too big and becoming bigger than others. In their minds, there was no question but that the *Schlaraffenland* was a world of big people and that the biggest of them all held the position of king.[58] They were also convinced that this wonderland had no thin inhabitants, for thin people would have had to leave it right away. The first response of young people to the preceding description was to say that people who do nothing grow big.

> That's really dumb because whoever doesn't work gets big, and whoever sleeps in gets big, too. (BD 14–16)
>
> Aha! You get totally big there. (GT 11–13)
>
> So people want to get big. (BT 14–16)

These young people have internalized the notion that being socially lazy is associated with being too big. As with the first part of the *Schlaraffenland* tale, they understood this section as a contrasting fantasy world and commented on it from their perspective. Consider first how the young people judged that this place was one where people are supposed to be lazy and are even rewarded for it. Did the young people disassociate themselves from such a picture of social order? Did they endorse the prevailing legitimations instead?

> I wouldn't go there in the first place; you die of boredom there. (GT 11–13)
>
> The fact that you're not allowed to work or do any sports—that's totally disgusting. (GT 14–16)
>
> Just that everybody's so lazy and dull. You can't do *anything* there. They're all so zapped. That's not nice. (GT 14–16)

In all group discussions, there was consensus among the young people that they would not desire a world in which they were not permitted to do anything. While they would find it attractive not to have to attend school and to be allowed to sleep in, it would bore them after a few days. They would like to be active and do something.

> I'm one who needs a day where I can be really lazy, but I can't lie in bed seven days at a time. That just doesn't work. (GD 14–16)

> OK, I'm fat. People think I don't get any exercise, but quite honestly, if I couldn't work a bit, if I were just to sit the whole time in front of the computer or ... sleep in for a long time, there wouldn't be anything left of my day. (BT 11–13)

It was important for the young people to underline that they reject this fantasy world. They spurned it as a possible objective social reality and legitimated social order. They added that they personally would not fit in there at all. They could not be lazy.

A similar result emerges from an analysis of the value young people attached to the second inversion of social legitimations. Would they approve of a social hierarchy that privileges those who achieve nothing?

> If someone is crowned king of the lazy, I'd find it actually totally stupid. (BD 14–16)
>
> It doesn't really make sense to have the laziest person be king. Because he's not hard working and can't be, he wouldn't do a thing and would still be named king. (GT 11–13)

The young people criticized the *Schlaraffenland* for having the "laziest" person assume the highest social position. Instead, they defended the purposefulness of assigning social positions based on merit and honoring people with social recognition if they meet expected standards.

The outcome was comparable for the third reversed legitimation: the social exclusion of those who were industrious. More than anything, the bigger young people wished to belong and not be excluded.[59] The fantasy of the *Schlaraffenland* offers the chance of being front and center in the crowd without having to do anything. Would the bigger young people nevertheless like to leave that place?

> F: I would leave it voluntarily.
> C: Me, too. Or I'd work so that they throw me out. (BD 14–16)
> E: I think the only positive thing about it is the final sentence.
> K: Yes, if someone . . .
> C: If someone is too hard working, . . .
> K: He has to leave the land. (GT 14–16)

Again, the relatively big young people declared their agreement with the dominant social order. They wanted to leave the *Schlaraffenland* and preferred to live in actual objective social reality. They welcomed the fact that social participation and integration stem primarily from work. By contrast, the *Schlaraffenland* represented to them a deviant social order that they rejected and did not want to belong to.

To summarize the issue thus far, the relatively big young people unmistakably distanced themselves from all three inversions of the prevailing social legitimations, explaining their perspective by contrasting the explanations and justifications governing the *Schlaraffenland* with those of actual society. Although the fairytale land offered them the option of a social order in which they faced no threat of being branded as nonconformists and deviators, they did not buy into it at all. Without hesitation, they unconditionally defended the received social order of the real world against that of the *Schlaraffenland*.

The fact that the young people were eager to portray themselves as conforming to the prevailing social order and as avoiding any deviance from it was not a surprising response to the way society deals with them. Nevertheless, we should note that the way they presented themselves cannot be taken for granted. It required them to commit themselves heavily to the dominant legitimations. For one thing, the participants in the group discussions were pubescent young people who were likely to be swayed by the fantasy world of the *Schlaraffenland* if only out of an adolescent desire to be provocative. A few spontaneous comments they made met these expectations: "cool" (BD 11–13), "I want to go there" (BT 11–13), "Boy, I'd be king" (GD 14–16). Scarcely uttered, these deviations from the official definition of reality were immediately rejected by the other young people. For another thing, the relatively big young people felt they had constantly experienced their affirmation of the social order failed to be noticed. They do not see themselves as deviants, but they nonetheless report being treated as such. As far as they are concerned, there are, thus, good reasons to doubt the authority of the social order, which evidently does not extend to them. Yet they do not repudiate that order at all. Instead, they stress that legitimations are objectively available and subjectively plausible to them.

This aspect calls for further explanation. Thus far, the young people's comments on the three inversions of the established legitimations have been analyzed more or less in separate groups. I now follow Berger and Luckmann in looking at the integration of the three legitimations into a "symbolic universe".[60] Were the young people persuaded by the inversions of the *Schlaraffenland*? Do they judge the social order described there as inherently consistent and coherent? In short, the answers are "no." The respondents said that the fantasy social order was a "poor system" (BT 11–13) and criticized its lack of "proper rules" (GT 11–13). Many of the young people discussed the imagined meaning of the *Schlaraffenland* in detail. In group discussion, they repeatedly came to the same conclusion: that this world is absurd and logically unsound.

> If there really is such a place and thin people were there, too, they would also make fun of the king. Then they'd say, "Look, that's the biggest one. He sleeps the longest and has the least energy." It's not good, either, if he's the king. Actually, it's only good if you are thrown out. (GD 11–13)
>
> Hey, look. As king you're big, too, so you can be laughed at. Thin people can laugh at him because he can't decide things for them. They can laugh at him because he's only the king of the big, not of the thin people. (GD 11–13)

The *Schlaraffenland* was absurd and fallacious in their view because it was inconceivable that the big inhabitants could ever rule over the thin ones. Even a "big *king*" would never be accepted by "thin subjects." The experience of the big young people has been that objective social reality clearly differentiates between thin and big individuals and that this distinction is legitimated by the social order. The social order sets the world of thin people apart from that of big ones and places them in a hierarchy. The young people have learned that this arrangement enjoys absolute acceptance and is immutable. The young people found it utterly unimaginable that society could see or treat thinness or fatness as anything beyond right or wrong, socially normal or socially deviant. The official definition of reality, they concluded, will always identify them as deviants.

To the comparatively big young participants in my study, objective social reality represented an overwhelmingly powerful and consistently "logical" context of meaning with which they portrayed themselves as conformists, at least if it had been reconstructed from those institutions and legitimations that turn the *Schlaraffenland* into its opposite. In other words, they strive to demonstrate that they neither reject these legitimations nor have to be brought back into the social order. Moreover, during the group discussions they showed no interest at all in the invitation "to fantasize" whether and how, from their perspective, the social order should change. They were intent on affirming their conformity.

Power of legitimate orders

Notably, the young people in the study made fewer changes and hedges in their statements about legitimations of the social order than they did in those about the order of eating. One reason for this outcome could be that they were able to communicate their affirmation of the social order directly. Although they had learned that society equates obesity with being lazy and that they themselves had done so as well, it seemed simpler for them to disassociate themselves from society's attribution of nonconformity with prevailing legitimations by stating that the legitimations were objectively available and subjectively plausible.

As for the order of eating, they have learned that society evaluates their bodies as a document of deviance from the norms, which is why these young people declare their acceptance of this social perception. Accordingly, the transcripts of the study frequently show formulations such as "though you can't tell from the way I look." At the same time, their emphasis on their acceptance of the order of eating and their familiarity with the "right dietary knowledge" presumably diverge a good deal from their everyday practices. The consequence is that the power inherent in the order of eating, namely, its acceptance as binding, frequently compels these young people to negate themselves. One can see from this response to the exercise of power through the establishment of a socially binding order of eating is not confined to labeling an individual an "actual or potential deviator." It is not just a matter of that person's stigmatization. It also goes further than that individual having to confirm that legitimations are objectively available to him or her and that they are subjectively plausible. The entire scope of that power is incomprehensible until one takes into account its attendant imperative as well: self-control to the point of self-negation. As this chapter reveals, the order of eating is interlinked with key parts of the social order. Indeed, they reinforce each other. A big body is taken as proof of deviance from both. Only by considering this perspective, too, can one understand the power of obesity.

Notes

1 See Eva Barlösius, *Soziologie des Essens: Eine sozial- und kulturwissenschaftliche Einführung in die Ernährungsforschung* (Weinheim: Juventa, 2011).

2 Margaret Mead, "Food and Feeding in Occupied Territory," *Public Opinion Quarterly* 7, no. 4 (1943): 618–28.

3 See Barlösius, *Soziologie des Essens*, 162–71.

4 Pierre Bourdieu, *Distinction: A Social Critique of the Judgement of Taste* (London: Routledge, 1984).

5 Gerhard J. Baudy, "Hierarchie oder: Die Verteilung des Fleisches," in *Neue Ansätze in der Religionswissenschaft*, ed. Burkhardt Gladegow and Hans G. Krippenberg (Munich: Kösel, 1983), 134.

6 Klaus Eder, *The Social Construction of Nature: A Sociology of Ecological Enlightenment*, trans. M. Ritter (London: Sage, 1996), 61.

7 See Peter L. Berger and Thomas Luckmann, *The Social Construction of Reality: A Treatise in the Sociology of Knowledge* (Garden City, NY: Anchor Books, [1966] 1991).

8 See Abigail C. Saguy, *What's with Fat?* (Oxford: Oxford University Press, 2013).

9 See Émile Durkheim, *Les règles de la méthode sociologique* (1985; Paris: Presses Universitaires de France, 1950).

10 I speak of "being big," "relatively big people," "getting bigger," and "somewhat bigger" because this article draws on results from a research project involving "relatively big" young people who used these words when referring to themselves. By adopting their own vocabulary, I hope to minimize any notion of denigration it might convey (see Eva Barlösius and Axel Philipps, "Felt Stigma and Obesity: Introducing the Generalized Other," *Social Science & Medicine* 130 (2015): 12, accessed May 20, 2016, doi:10.1016/j.socscimed.2015.01.048.)

11 See Eva Barlösius, *Dicksein: Wenn der Körper das Verhältnis zur Gesellschaft bestimmt* (Frankfurt/M.: Campus, 2014).

12 This response reflects that the body appears to have become associated with everything signifying a "good life" (see Mike Featherstone, "The Body in Consumer Culture," in *The Body: Social Process and Cultural Theory*, ed. Mike Featherstone et al. (London: Sage, 1991), 186.

13 Gerhard J. Baudy, "Hierarchie oder: Die Verteilung des Fleisches. Eine ethologische Studie über die Tischordnung als Wurzel sozialer Organisation, mit besonderer Berücksichtigung der altgriechischen Gesellschaft," in *Neue Ansätze in der Religionswissenschaft*, ed. Burkhardt Gladigow and Henning G. Kippenberg (Munich: Kösel, 1983), 131–74.

14 Eva Barlösius, *Naturgemäße Lebensführung: Zur Geschichte der Lebensreform um die Jahrhundertwende* (Frankfurt/M.: Campus, 1997).

15 See Mackert in this volume.

16 Puhl and Heuer reviewed more than two hundred publications: Rebecca M. Puhl and Chelsea A. Heuer, "The Stigma of Obesity: A Review and Update," *Obesity* 17, no. 5 (2009): 941–64. Other important studies are Tatiana Andreyeva et al., "Changes in Perceived Weight Discrimination among Americans, 1995–1996 through 2004–2006," *Obesity* 16, no. 5(2008): 1129–34; Regina F. Bento et al., "The Stigma of Obesity and Discrimination in Performance Appraisal: A Theoretical Model," *International Journal of Human Resource Management* 23, no. 15 (2012): 3196–224; Leanne Joanisse and Anthony Synnott, "Fighting Back: Reactions and Resistance to the Stigma of Obesity," in *Interpreting Weight: The Social Management of Fatness and Thinness*, ed. Donna Maurer and Jeffery Sobal (Hawthorne/New York: Aldine, 1999); Sophie Lewis et al., "How Do Obese Individuals Perceive and Respond to the Different Types of Obesity Stigma That They Encounter in Their Daily Lives? A Qualitative Study," *Social Science & Medicine* 73, no. 9 (2011): 1349–56, and Dianne Neumark-Sztainer et al., "Weight-Teasing among Adolescents: Correlations with Weight Status and Disordered Eating Behaviors," *International Journal of Obesity* 26, no. 1 (2002): 123–31.

17 Nancy E. Adler and Judith Stewart, "Reducing Obesity: Motivating Action While Not Blaming the Victim," *Milbank Quarterly* 87, no. 1 (2009): 51.

18 Puhl and Heuer, "Stigma."

19 Allison James, "Embodied Being(s), Understanding the Self and the Body in Childhood," in *The Body, Childhood and Society*, ed. Alan Prout (London: Palgrave Macmillan, 2000); I. Solbes and I. Enesco, "Explicit and Implicit Anti-fat Attitudes in Children and Their Relationships with Their Body Images," *Obesity Facts* 3, no. 1 (2010): 23–32; Petra Warschburger, "Psychosoziale Faktoren der Adipositas in Kindheit und Adoleszenz," in *Handbuch Essstörungen und Adipositas*, ed. Stephan Herpertz et al. (Berlin/Heidelberg: Springer, 2008).

20 As reported by Wei Su and Aurelia Di Santo, "Preschool Children's Perceptions of Overweight Peers," *Journal of Early Childhood Research* 10, no. 1 (2012): 20.

21 Audrey L. MacNevin, "Embodying Sociological Mindfulness: Learning about Social Inequality through the Body," *Teaching Sociology*, 32, no. 3 (2004): 315.

22 Kwan calls it "body privilege": Samantha Kwan, "Navigating Public Spaces: Gender, Race, and Body Privilege in Everyday Life," *Feminist Formations* 22, no. 2 (2010): 144–66.

23 Actually, yet another aspect is required, too—that of social inequalities; see Barlösius, *Dicksein*.

24 Berger and Luckmann, *Social Construction*.

25 Berger and Luckmann, *Social Construction*, 77.

26 Ibid., 59.

27 Ibid., 61.

28 Ibid., 92.

29 Ibid., 110.

30 Ibid.

31 Another function of legitimations is to enable the individual to describe his or her life trajectory as "subjectively meaningful."

32 Berger and Luckmann, *Social Construction*, 113.

33 Ibid.

34 This study is based on a project funded by the German Federal Ministry of Education and Research and entitled "Improvement in the Effectiveness of Obesity Prevention for Socially Disadvantaged Children and Youth—Targeted Strategies to Enhance the Health-Related Resources for Encouraging Responsibility for Diet and Exercise" (01E0813). All results are presented in Barlösius, *Dicksein*.

35 The "World Café" is a method that facilitates open discussions on a given subject, in order to access the "collective intelligence" of a group of experts.

36 The group discussions took place in the fall of 2009.

37 Ralf Bohnsack, "Gruppendiskussionsverfahren und Milieuforschung," in *Handbuch Qualitative Forschungsmethoden in der Erziehungswissenschaft*, ed. Barbara Friebertshäuser and Annedore Prengel (Weinheim/

Munich: Juventa, 1997); Peter Loos and Burkhard Schäffer, *Das Gruppendiskussionsverfahren* (Opladen: Springer VS, 2001); Serge Moscovici and Willem Doise, *Dissensions et consensus: Une théorie générale des décisions collectives* (Paris: Presses Universitaires de France, 1992).

38 Berger and Luckmann, *Social Construction*, chap. 2.

39 Of lower class children, 12.33% are categorized as obese, though only 5% of middle-class children are obese (Marcel Helbig and Stefanie Jähnen, "Bildungsbenachteiligt durch Übergewicht: Warum adipöse Kinder in der Schule schlechter abschneiden," *Zeitschrift für Soziologie* 42 (2013): Online Appendix, V).

40 For details on recruitment for the study, see Barlösius, *Dicksein*, 39–45. The parents of the young people signed a letter of consent, and anonymity was guaranteed.

41 The project compared German and Turkish children and teenagers because the prevalence of Turkish adolescents being obese (13.50%) is high compared to German young people (5.5%).

42 Clear differences emerged regarding other aspects of the group discussions, especially those concerning matters of everyday practice, such as apparel, leisure time, meals, and desires for the future. Divergence along the lines of German or Turkish background was small among the boys. It was far greater among the girls. The Turkish girls, for example, stood out for their very high educational aspirations. They spoke little about their own leisure activities, being heavily involved in family and household responsibilities instead. Moreover, they complained that their eating behavior was monitored by their fathers and brothers. For details, see Barlösius, *Dicksein*.

43 Alfred Schütz and Thomas Luckmann, *The Structures of the Life-World, vol. 2* (Evanston, IL: Northwestern University Press, [1979] 1989).

44 Schütz and Luckmann, *Structures*, vol. 2, 120.

45 Dieter Richter, *Schlaraffenland: Geschichte einer populären Phantasie* (Cologne: Eugen Diederichs Verlag, 1984).

46 For additional literature on places like Big Rock Candy Mountain as a social utopia, see Miguel Pina E. Cunha, "Dreaming of Cockaigne: Individual Fantasies of the Perfect Workplace," *FEUNL Working Paper* 414 (2002), accessed May 23, 2016, http://fesrvsd.fe.unl.pt/WPFEUNL/WP2002/wp414.pdf; Hans-Jörg Gilomen, "Das Schlaraffenland und andere Utopien im Mittelalter," *Basler Zeitschrift für Geschichte und Altertumskunde* 104 (2004): 213–48; Caspar Gottschling, *Der Staat Von Schlaraffen-Land* (Hanover: Wehrhahn, 2007); Frederick B. Jonassen, "Lucian's 'Saturanlia', the Land of Cockaigne, and the Mummers' Plays," *Folklore* 101, no. 1 (1990): 58–68; and Frank H. Ross, "An Interpretation of Land of Cockaigne (1567) by Pieter Breugel the Elder," *Sixteenth Century Journal* 22, no. 2 (1991): 299–329.

47 See Martin Müller, *Das Schlaraffenland: Der Traum von Faulheit und Müßiggang* (Vienna: Edition Brandstätter, 1984): 13.

48 Brüder Grimm, Kinder- und Haus-Märchen (Berlin: Realschulbuchandlung, 1812).

49 Herman Pleij, *Der Traum vom Schlaraffenland: Mittelalterliche Phantasien vom vollkommenen Leben* (Frankfurt/M.: Fischer, 1997): 444.

50 Cunha, "Dreaming," 3, showed that the basic motifs in the tale are understood even when it is unknown, for they evoke analogies to the present.

51 Barlösius, *Soziologie des Essens*, 19–21; Pleij, *Traum vom Schlaraffenland*; Richter, *Schlaraffenland*; Werner Wunderlich, "Das Schlaraffenland in der deutschen Sprache und Literatur: Bibliographischer Überblick über den Forschungsstand," *Fabula* 27 (1986): 54–74.

52 Wunderlich, "Schlaraffenland", 65.

53 See Müller, *Schlaraffenland*, 24.

54 Richter, *Schlaraffenland*, 10 and 17.

55 The quotations are excerpts from the group discussions. The language in some of the quotations has been corrected to improve their comprehensibility, but neither the substance nor the manner of expression has been altered. In the transcripts, B stands for boy; G, for girl; T, for Turkish; and D, for German. The numerals give the age ranges. Each participant was also assigned a code letter to show that different persons were speaking. With few exceptions, however, the speaker's identity is not important in the analysis, so I have generally deleted these tags for the sake of legibility. They appear only in discussion sequences to indicate exchanges between two or more persons.

56 See Jane Wardle et al., "Depression in Adolescent Obesity: Cultural Moderators of the Association between Obesity and Depression Symptoms," *International Journal of Obesity* 30 (2006): 634–43; Margaret D. Hanson and Edith Chen, "Socioeconomic Status, Race, and Body Mass Index: The Mediating Role of Physical Activity and Sedentary Behaviors during Adolescence," *Journal of Pediatric Psychology* 32, no. 3 (2007): 250–9.

57 Eva Barlösius, Alexandra von Garmissen, and Grit Voigtmann, *Dicksein—über die gesellschaftliche Erfahrung dick zu sein*. Leibniz Universität, Hanover, December 18, 2012, accessed May 23, 2016, https://www.ish.uni-hannover.de/fileadmin/soziologie/pdf/allgemein/leibinz-uni-hannover_studie_dicksein_RZ.pdf; Barlösius, *Dicksein*.

58 The young people knew neither the German fairy tale about *Schlaraffenland* nor the corresponding oil painting created by Pieter Breugel the Elder (1525/30–1569) around 1567. For them, the connection with laziness and fatness therefore did not stem from literature or visual art but rather from daily experience.

59 See Barlösius, von Garmissen, and Voigtmann, *Dicksein—Über die gesellschaftliche Erfahrung*.

60 Berger and Luckmann, *Social Construction*, 92.

8

When the grease runs through the paper: On the consumption of ultragreasy bureks

Jernej Mlekuž

Before the paper gets greasy

The burek, an important, frequently prepared dish among many immigrants to Slovenia and their descendants, is probably also Slovenia's most popular fast food.[1] This pie, made of phyllo dough and filled with meat, cheese, vegetables, fruits, and various other mixed fillings, was brought to Slovenian towns in the 1960s by Albanian burek makers from Macedonia—the owners of street burek kiosks, who offered some of the rare, and in many places the only fast food available at night during the ascetic socialist times. In the mid-1990s, this urban street hero reached deep into the Slovenian dietary mainstream. As various newspaper surveys indicate, and as a quick stroll through the city streets would show you, it is the winner in the fast food or street food category. But today the burek is no longer found only on city streets and in the kitchens of immigrant (and increasingly also "nonimmigrant") families. It is now stealing shelf space from other deep-frozen items in the freezers of (super)markets—it is produced in frozen and nonfrozen form by both of Slovenia's largest industrial bakeries as well as a plethora of smaller bakeries. It is eaten by the Slovenian armed forces, enjoyed as a snack in Slovenian schools (although, owing to its nutritional "inappropriateness," not more than once a month), gets served at numerous formal and informal parties and events, takes to the air on some flights of Slovenia's national airline, and rides in trucks carrying Slovenian goods to foreign markets. And since 2013, it can be purchased with a filling made of Carniolan sausage (the flagship of Slovene cuisine) under the name *kranjski* (Carniolan) *burek*.[2] (Carniola was a central, and the most "Slovenian," part of the Austro-Hungarian Empire, and the adjective is now used to grace many things that are considered to be Slovenian par excellence).[3]

However, the burek has not just conquered Slovenian streets, schools, shops, kitchens, and numerous other public and private places and nonplaces but has also grease-stained the Slovene language. Today it has a privileged place in Slovenia as a loaded metaphor for immigrants, Southerners, the Balkans, and the former federal republic and the phenomena associated with it. The burek is probably the best-known and most widely discussed and problematized immigrant in Slovenia. This is made clear by the best-known Slovenian nationalist graffito, *burek, nein danke*. It is also, to a great extent, an assimilated immigrant in Slovenia (e.g., the Carniolan burek). Moreover, it has become in a way the most convenient representative or signifier of unhealthy and greasy food. Without the burek, which seems to be enjoyed in the language much more than on the palate, it would be difficult to conceive of not just the thoughtscape of Slovenian nationalism but also the rhetorical arsenal of promoters of healthy lifestyles and health food.

The *Lonely Planet* guide to the Slovenian capital, Ljubljana, provides the "greasy lowdown" on the burek. It is increasingly referred to as "greasy junk food" in all sorts of "healthy-lifestyle" texts in Slovenia, and it is occasionally the object of true worship among certain rebellious teenage groups—in the words of an adherent, "the burek is great" (a paraphrase of *Allahu akbar*).[4] But as I will show in this chapter, this teenage fight, this disobedience, this rebellion has to be understood as more than simply a war of ideas, concepts, discourses, and ideologies. It is more accurately an explicit rebellion against a healthy-lifestyle discourse—a discourse that insinuates that we must live healthily and correctly and that marks this "Slovenian" street hero as a lowlife. I take seriously Marshall Sahlins's observation that power today is an "intellectual black hole into which all kinds of cultural contents get sucked."[5] And it would seem that research on civil disobedience has been particularly sucked into this "intellectual black hole." According to Per Hergren it has been transformed through numerous interpretive devices into one of the most flexible, elastic, and adaptable of concepts.[6] The research into civil disobedience has been subject to criticism owing to both its fetishization[7] and its romanticization.[8] Lila Abu-Lughod thus warns that much research on everyday civil disobedience does not succeed in being anything more than a heroic paean to rebels. In her opinion, researchers omit a critical issue, that of complex interactions, relations, and unequal relationships. In this chapter,

I take a further step in the problematizing of civil disobedience. I show the place of civil disobedience within the story of teenage consumption of "ultragreasy" bureks, which I investigated through conversations with secondary-school students and through direct observation in 2006 and 2007. To put it slightly differently, I look at how disobedience and power are articulated in the wider social and material context in concrete dietary practices. But first, I examine in greater detail the role and place of the burek within healthy-lifestyle and medical discourse, and particularly its intimate relationship with greasiness.

Greasy junk food

According to theoreticians of late modernity, the current high level of attention to the body, health, and nutrition can be understood as an individualized response to increasingly complex social activities, which drive the individual away from political and social decisions.[9] The individual's focus on his or her body, health, and nutrition is therefore a move into the apparently manageable individual sphere, while at the same time being a social, "public" presentation of individual responsibility to the self and to the wider society, which at the societal level appears (and is judged) by indicators of a(n) (un)healthy body.[10] As Anthony Giddens says, "We have become responsible for the design of our own bodies."[11]

During the twentieth century, medicine developed into a highly sophisticated system of social control, which has not only transformed economic and political issues into individual issues but also, to an even greater extent, taken over areas that were once the province of religious and legal institutions. As Kevin White explains, "activities that were once thought of as immoral and the domain of the Church (e.g. gluttony), or the law (e.g. suicide) are now seen as medical issues."[12] Medicine, or medical discourse, which is among the most dominant in modern Western societies, has permeated not only popular, lifestyle-related, media, and other discourses but also the sphere of everyday life.[13] The medicalization of everyday practices, according to White, poses the question of whether we truly wish to medicalize every aspect of our lives—our personalities, love lives, marriages, children.[14] Here we might ask whether we have merely posed the question, or whether the answers have been imposed on us.[15]

One of these questions, which most often imposes unavoidable responses, has to do with the avoidance or fear of fat. Fats, particularly animal fats, once a highly valued component of food,[16] have, at least recently, taken on the status of an "evil substance" within professional and popular discourse.[17] As studies carried out in Western (post)industrial societies have shown, people routinely label greasy food as unhealthy, particularly if the fats are visible.[18]

In my book *Burek: A Culinary Metaphor,* I showed that greasiness is one of the dominant and most common connotations of the burek, and probably the most dominant in the society of those who emphasize its material and physiological characteristics.[19] Furthermore, the burek has become a signifier, which is frequently, if not most often, used when people in Slovenia write, speak, and think about greasiness. The greasiness of the burek is therefore the point around which healthy-lifestyle discourse circles, particularly when it addresses the burek in a fictive, imaginative, and notional sense. And of course the burek's greasiness does not escape the attention of professional and scientific discourse. In an excerpt from a diploma thesis entitled "The Meat Burek in Nutrition: An Analysis of Quality and Proposal for Improvement," the author first and foremost reprimands the burek for its greasiness: "A comparison of the chemical content and the results of sensory analysis of the homemade sample with the other samples indicates the possibility of a better product with respect to the selection and reduced proportion of *fats,*[20] reduced proportion of added NaCl and increased proportion of meat."[21]

While the high proportion of fats in the burek is why the food is condemned in scientific and professional nutritional discourse, this same condemnation is even more predominant in unprofessional, popular discourse.[22] When evaluating bureks, "an ordinary guy, but also a major burekologist," as Franc "Lanko" Marušič describes himself, continually mentions, assesses, and evaluates their greasiness. On the *Delo* website, in the "Burek blog," where we find these assessments, he states the following: "The idea is simple. The quality of bureks in burek shops varies widely. The price not so much. After every burek I eat, I will write in this blog what it was like. How greasy, how tasty, the shape, the price, etc."[23] Thus, greasiness is positioned before taste. Numerous interviewees, interlocutors, and friends who have told me that they do not eat bureks or eat them only rarely, most often gave greasiness as the reason. This is the reason offered most often, and without me even asking them about greasiness. For example, one interviewee, replying by e-mail to the question "Do you have any other comments regarding 'the burek' and 'subcultures', regarding 'the burek' and 'Slovenian culture', or regarding the burek in general?" replied succinctly, "Yes. I think the burek is too *greasy.*"[24] The greasiness of the burek also frequently stains everyday life. Actually, we usually try not to let it, as we read in the online diary of a blogger named Mika titled "(I Don't Know What's Going) On":

> "Come on over. I hope you haven't eaten."
>
> "We'll go get a burek at the station," I said, laughing.
>
> "Yeah, right. Bureks are way too greasy. That's the first reason against them. And the second is obviously some dirty stand at the station. No thanks."[25]

Browsing the Internet merely confirms the indelibility of the burek's greasiness. On the website SMSdiete.si, in a discussion about food separation (the notion that fats, hydrocarbons, and lipids should be consumed separately), Afrodita responds to emanuelina's question of whether she can eat a cheese burek: "Given that things have to be separated, I believe that a cheese burek is not exactly the right thing plus it's greasy as lightning so I would avoid it!"[26] In a comment by Gomi on Marin Medak's blog entitled "How Can Youth Be Motivated to Have an Active Lifestyle?" we read the following: "We are too fat due to the quality of our food and our way of eating.... A greasy burek is cheaper faster and usually even better prepared than grilled fish."[27] While we are on the subject of fish, on the website Ribiči Slovenije (Fishermen of Slovenia) in the "Kraparski forum" (Carp fisher's forum), in a debate entitled "Catch-release areas for carp a thing of the past?", the burek leaves the following grease stains: "Someone mentioned bureks, and asked if we were so poor that we couldn't afford them. I would just like to say that a burek/fast food is significantly less healthy than a fresh-caught trout! I would recommend that he add fish to his diet at least once a week, instead of poisoning his circulatory system with greasy bureks."[28] In a debate entitled "Do you eat bureks??" on the website Genspot, slepiurar (blind watchmaker) asks, "do they still sell that *greasy* filth?"[29] And since January 2013, there has been a group on Facebook called Mastni burek (Greasy burek), which mainly features advertisements for various food products.

Greasiness is also a very frequent element of various media statements on bureks. In an article with the suggestive/scary headline "Tiger Tamers Behind the School Benches," young people are advised, "In order to acquire all of these characteristics, exercise and proper nutrition are very important (you have to eat healthy food, and give up fried steaks, French fries, bureks and other greasy and sweet junk foods."[30] In a column entitled "Verifying Rumors" in the gossip magazine *Nova*, an article entitled "[TV presenter and actress] Katarina Čas. Lover of Bureks and Tripe" begins thusly,

> This beauty doesn't just eat salads and low-calorie fat-free meals but also occasionally allows herself a greasy burek. "I definitely have a burek at least twice a month," said the television host, who eats them when she does not have a lot of time for lunch. "The next day I eat more vegetables."[31]

On the back cover of the first anthology of comics by artists from Eastern and Central Europe entitled *Stripburek: Comics from Behind the Rusty Iron Curtain*, a special thematic issue of the Slovenian comic strip magazine *Stripburger*, we find an equation with the burek's greasiness squared (Figure 8.1).[32]

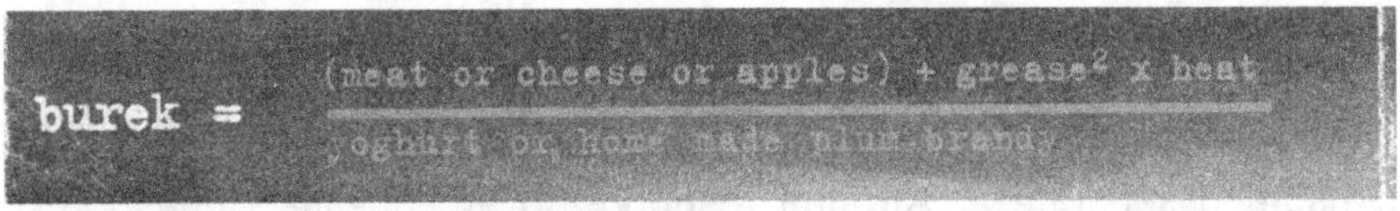
burek =
(meat or cheese or apples) + grease² x heat
yoghurt or home made plum brandy

FIGURE 8.1 *Burek equation. Jakob Klemenčič and Marcel Ruijters, first published in Stripburek——Comics from Behind the Rusty Iron Curtain, 1997. Courtesy Stripburger/Forum Ljubljana.*

In an article entitled "The Clothes Make the Soldier," which talks about the new uniforms for the Slovenian armed forces, we read the following: "The materials are a story unto themselves: the jacket, trousers and skirt are made of Teflon-coated wool and polyester, which is waterproof and oil-resistant. This means that it is highly resistant to stains, which is particularly welcome when snacking on a *greasy burek*."[33] In the words of Roland Barthes, "Food . . . is not only a collection of products that can be used for statistical or nutritional studies. It is also, and at the same time, a system of communication, a body of images, a protocol of usages, situations and behavior."[34]

But healthy-lifestyle discourse has not only bit into the world of the media, where it could chew on greasy bureks forever. It has also feasted on, or more precisely, greased up burek production. Nearly all commercial producers of bureks as well as noncommercial burek makers have told me that they have in one way or another reduced or at least attempted to reduce the fat content. This has taken the form of changes to the filling (e.g., low-fat cottage cheese or meat), or to the oil or the type of fat used (e.g., vegetable oil instead of lard).[35] To this degreasing of the burek we could add the recipe for a "low-fat sirov burek" made of whole wheat phyllo dough (which we can buy, according to the recipe, at Hofer, an Austrian, i.e., Western, supermarket chain), with unpasteurized light cottage cheese, (cottage cheese 0.9% milk fat), two eggs and no other fats (listed). The recipe is posted on the website Maxximum portal, whose mission is to "provide knowledge about sports and healthy nutrition, fitness and bodybuilding" and whose slogan is "Dedicated to a fit philosophy." This slice of burek comes with 329.5 calories, containing 32.5 g of protein, 34.1 g of carbohydrates, and 6.4 g of fat.[36] Pedantic and healthy, right?

Here we have to deal with Michel Foucault's ideas of "regimes of truth" and " 'general politics' of truth: that is, the types of discourse which [society] accepts and makes function as true."[37] Truth, knowledge, or as is most apt when talking about the greasiness of the burek, self-evidence, as Foucault states, "isn't outside power."[38] Discourses have a unique power to define and constitute objects of knowledge, and a sinister power to erase and divide. Discourses spread, introduce, confirm, and establish certain meanings, knowledge, and truths, and nullify, silence, and erase others. We are subject to the establishment of truth via authority. Authority can therefore not be exercised without the production of truth, self-evidence, and knowledge. Healthy-lifestyle discourse, dedicated to the "philosophy of healthy living," tells us every day in the media, in conversations, in supermarket freezers that the burek is a low-down, greasy junk food. And not only that. It also suggests and not infrequently imposes ways of handling greasy junk food, changes (chews on) it, and limits and stigmatizes it. Power constitutes bodies, behaviors, thoughts, and feelings, and at the same time, it controls and shapes them.

Of course, the burek is not just greasy. It is, as we have seen in numerous burek statements, (therefore) also unhealthy.[39] In the aforementioned debate entitled "Do You Eat Bureks??" on the website Genspot, the aforementioned blind watchmaker enters the debate thusly: "steps: ... burek .... doctor's office .... Petra Držaj [Ljubljana hospital] .... žale [Ljubljana cemetery]."[40] Pop singer and pianist Neisha, in a supplement to the daily *zurnal24* called "Celebrity Diets," gives a succinct answer to the question "What do you like to eat?" She answers, "My favorites are the things I shouldn't eat. I love a good burek at four in the morning." In a promotional invitation to visit Slovenia in the guide *Via Stansted Express*, which is put out on the train seats for Ryanair passengers traveling from Stansted Airport to London, in addition to various exhortations to visit pleasant Ljubljana coffeehouses, the town market, and bars and clubs, "Britons are invited to have a midday snack of burek, a local specialty made with cheese, which they can buy on the street. But it's not for people with weak hearts."[41] Most often the burek seems to be understood as unhealthy: as "things I shouldn't eat," and "not for people with weak hearts." This is precisely because it is greasy. In one of his evaluations, the aforementioned burek assessor Lanko says, "Since [the burek] was not too greasy, I can say that it was one of the healthiest."[42]

Medical or healthy-lifestyle discourse has thus discovered in the burek's greasiness its Achilles heel, and has directed the majority of its spear toward it. Greasiness, that demonic quality of the new, healthy-lifestyle-oriented age, has been detected in the burek, and this has led to a pogrom, an inquisition, a witch hunt with all the attendant spectacle. Such greasy burek statements could be served up forever. But let us go back to young people and their eating of ultragreasy bureks.

When the grease runs through the paper

Numerous studies have shown that children and teenagers often use food to establish their personal autonomy and as a means of resistance against the authority of adults.[43] Food, particularly fast food, is one of the great battlefields on which wars are fought between parents and children, between the old and the young. Food, of course, divides parents and children on several levels. Parents and adults discipline (or at least attempt to discipline) children and young people with food and thus establish authority.[44]

As Claude Fischler says, for parents, "control over the child's diet is vital. Not only is the offspring's present health at stake, but his whole future evolution, his entire person."[45] We can also see the special status of children's food in nutritional ideology, in which children's and young people's favorite dishes usually have low nutritional status.[46] It is precisely this low status of children's dishes, according to Allison James, that, in addition to taste, is the reason for the popularity of these dishes among children and youth: "Adult order is manipulated so that what adults esteem is made to appear ridiculous; what adults despise is invested with prestige."[47]

It was on this battlefield between the old and the young that the battle for the burek's meanings was (and probably still is being) fought. But it seems that we also have to deal with other streams of disobedience. Certain groups of male Ljubljana secondary schoolers, mainly or exclusively from high schools, use the symbolic and conspicuous consumption of greasy bureks as a form of rebellion against the dominant healthy-lifestyle discourse with which they are bombarded in the media, in advertising, and in formal and informal educational settings. As Foucault says, "discourse is not simply that which translates struggles or systems of domination, but is the thing for which and by which there is struggle, discourse is the power which is to be seized."[48]

As a study of the nutritional habits of Ljubljana elementary school students showed, "students are well acquainted with healthy lifestyles and nutrition and do not include fast food among healthy foods."[49] So they knew what they should not eat. For these students, particularly or exclusively groups of boys, not all bureks are equally good (or bad in a good way). The only good and proper bureks are greasy ones, which are usually made and sold on city streets by certain Albanian burek makers. Bureks that are considered less greasy, that is, bureks from "Slovenian" bakeries and industrial plants, are not considered good bureks. The ideal burek is therefore, as you can hear among secondary schoolers, an "ultragreasy burek" where the "grease runs through the paper." High school student A. J., who, as he admits, makes fun of dieting and counting calories, responds in an e-mail that "a greasier burek is usually better . . . when you get a burek that you can see through the paper, you already know it's going to be good."[50] High school student J. V. is even more to the point: "The definition of a burek is that it has to be greasy."[51] And it is not just direct statements that speak of this type of subversiveness of burek consumption. The eating of greasy bureks is often spiced with jokes at the expense of counting calories, obesity, women's avoidance of fatty foods and fattening foods in general, and at the expense of health. We list just a few of the statements by which I was inspired by the prolific J. V.,[52] and a few that I obtained by observing small groups of secondary schoolers while they were eating bureks on a spring afternoon in 2007 in front of the Ljubljana snack bar Dino Burek:

> "Hey, let's count calories."
>
> "One time my friend asked [a burek seller] for a diet burek. And I have no idea if he [the seller] got it."
>
> "I couldn't eat a whole burek, let's just take one. And there are five of us. [Laughter.] Two or three girls get one together. I chowed two by myself."
>
> "Those greasy bureks there [at a street burek stand] are not healthy, let's go to McDonald's, it's healthier."
>
> "I can't eat bureks, I'll get fat."

A group of students from Bežigrad High School who occasionally have bureks instead of school snacks, or enjoy a burek at a nearby burek bar after a difficult class, often make jokes at the expense of the female clerk. She supposedly only washes her hands once a week, and in this (not) washing is supposedly where the key to the greasiness of the burek resides: if she washes her hands on Thursday night, the bureks will be less greasy on Friday morning, but will be greasier each successive day after that.[53]

The burek thus plays the role among secondary school students that it was given by the healthy-lifestyle discourse—a signifier of greasiness, of greasy, unhealthy fast food—but it is no longer understood as exclusive and negative, but as approving and positive.[54] Fat, that demonic substance, that cornerstone of scandal, at least in the more fictive segment of healthy-lifestyle discourse, thus becomes among secondary schoolers a quality, which is talked about at full volume. Translated very freely from the semiotic language of Barthes: connotation is not just a tool of repression, an ideological illusion in the hands and possession of the rulers (in his opinion the bourgeoisie). Connotation is also an emancipating tool in the hands of the subjugated. It is a tool, a strategy that is available to everyone who is caught in a relationship of power, since power, according to Foucault, "is exercised only over free subjects, and only insofar as they are free."[55] Power is thus, as demonstrated by Foucault as well as by Edward Said and others, also productive.[56] It is not merely legal and negative. It speaks not only about what we may not do but is also technical and positive. It allows us to be able to do things. Foucault's frequent argument is that power only constructs that which is supposed to be the subject of repression.

However, the main role in this story of teenage burek eating, at least in my opinion, is played by the burek, and not by healthy-lifestyle discourse,

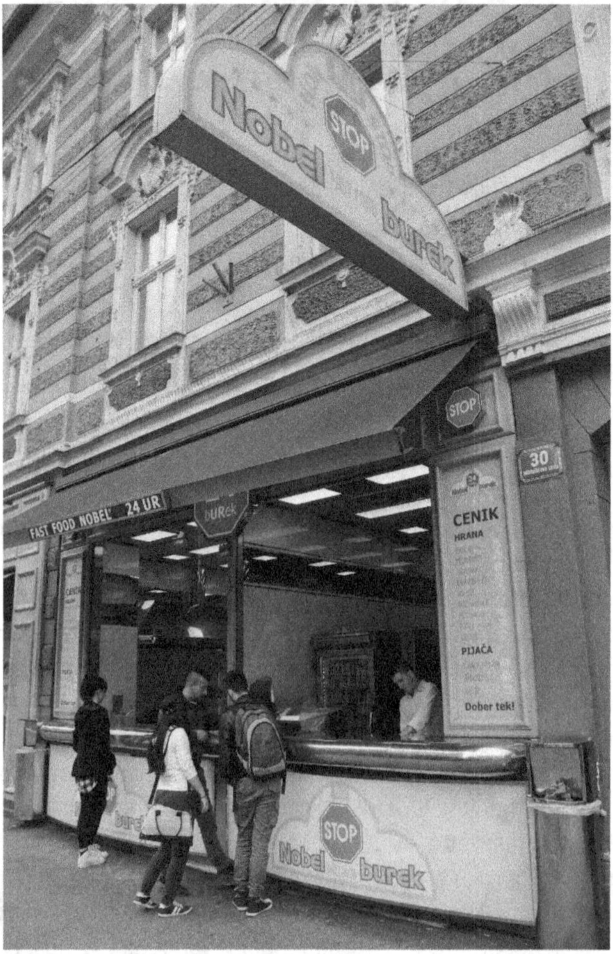

FIGURE 8.2 *The eating of greasy bureks. Photo © Jernej Mlekuž, Ljubljana 2015.*

high school rebellion, or signifying practice. But let us begin this story from a slightly different angle.

As Foucault maintains, power relations cannot exist without places of disobedience. "For," he writes, "if it is true that at the heart of power relations and as a permanent condition of their existence there is an insubordination and a certain essential obstinacy on the part of the principles of freedom, then there is no relationship of power without the means of escape or possible flight."[57] Disobedience and rebellion, as Dick Hebdige demonstrated using the example of British subcultures, are also implemented at the level of the everyday, involving apparently banal and insignificant things.[58] According to Hebdige, the subcultural challenge to the dominant culture does not arise directly from its opposition to it, but is reflected and manifested primarily at the level of style. In the case of teenage burek eating it seems that this rebellion is slightly more materialized or objectified. What do I mean by this materializing or objectification? I mean that this teenage rebellion or conspicuous consumption of greasy bureks cannot be understood primarily as a rebellion against the hegemonic ideas of healthy-lifestyle discourse in which the burek appears merely as a more or less random medium, a semiotic tool, a signifier. I believe that this high school rebellion (if it can be called rebellion) should be understood more as a rebellion with and for the burek, and not as a clear and planned rebellion against the dominant healthy-lifestyle discourse. Healthy-lifestyle discourse thus appears as a sort of appendage, a parasite on the popular—cheap, nearly always and everywhere available and filling—burek, which additionally conditions and colors the rebellion with and for the burek.[59] This is further corroborated by the conversations with burek-eating secondary school students, who only rarely and with difficulty perceive, recognize, and conceptualize the alleged great enemy, healthy-lifestyle discourse. M. Č., a friend and schoolmate of the author of the majority of the above statements, J. V., comments on his friend's humor and his connection with the burek as follows:

> Yeah, J. V. loves to do those kinds of things. And then we crack up. But at least in my case its usually just about making fun of girls who totally think they're fat and that they have to lose weight and all. And it's also about the fact that bureks are good. I didn't ever think about a rebellion against the media 'cause I usually don't even read those kinds of things and even when I do, they don't grab me.[60]

As Karl Marx would say, "We are not aware of this, nevertheless we do it."[61] The burek is, as I have said, a signifier of the dominant healthy-lifestyle discourse, an object of unwanted identity, a threat to the dominant health, thinness, and beauty-seeking world.[62] In this battle for the burek, some burek soldiers, that is, eaters of ultragreasy bureks, more or less consciously recognize the burek's enemy, that is, the social, cultural, and gendered emphasis on the thin and beautiful body. But, of course, it appears that generally speaking, jokes, gags, and humor are more important than any serious rebellion, high-minded ideals, or objectives. As Hebdige showed, subcultures cannot be understood as a direct rebellion against the dominant culture, hegemony, and consensus enforced by the authorities. The rebellion is manifested through spectacular style, which has to be understood, as Hebdige[63] indicated, as intentional communication—communication within subcultures, which is emphasized and unusual, which draws attention to itself, which presents, inverts, and destroys the dominant meanings and uses of commodities.[64] Of course, we have to read this intentional communication, at least in the case of teenage burek eating, primarily as intentional at the level of the subculture. But this certainly does not mean that it is done consciously and even understood by all of the individuals in the subculture. We probably have to put the word "rebellion" in quotation marks. According to Susan Seymour, we can only speak of rebellion in the case of conscious and intentional acts of opposition.[65] Rather than the problematic concept of rebellion, it is more appropriate to talk about a kind of zone, a space of teenage autonomy or at least a feeling of being unsupervised or of escape, as illustrated by this advice on eetaq.si or Fajn se 'mej! ("Have a Good One!")—"A teen website where kids learn things they don't teach at school, and which make their parents blush." Among the many pieces of advice given in response to "How to behave at the graduation ball? What is EETAQ [*itak*—self-evident, or in this case self-evidently cool], and what is IDIOTIC behavior?", we find in the third place on the list, that is, a very important place, the following suggestion:

> Go out for a burek—EETAQ!
>
> It is truly a festive evening, which your parents paid for with their entire fortune. But if a person dances and goes wild all night, at a certain point they're gonna get extra hungry. Or they opt for a short romantic trip for a burek in sympathetic company. There's nothing better than being a little mischievous, going for the alternative, and eating a burek in 300 euro clothes. But be careful not to spill. Cleaning up the grease stains could cost you more than the burek.[66]

Thus, in untangling this teenage conspicuous consumption and appropriation of the (ultra)greasy burek, I think we have to look for the beginning of the story in the burek's availability, affordability, quality of being very filling, and, of course, also or primarily in its superpopularity (Figure 8.3). Only afterward do the meanings, discourse, "rebellions" appear, which additionally flavor this consumption or appropriation. If we are already dealing with an analysis of power, then it is an analysis of power at its edges, in those places where it becomes, in Foucault's vocabulary, capillary, that is, an analysis of power outside of the legal rules, an analysis of the investment of power in institutions, embodied in various techniques and associations with the material circumstances. We have to deal, as anthropologist Sherry Ortner said, with "projects on the edge of power," or "cultural life 'on the margins of power' "[67]—"the workings of agency in context in which such relations [the workings of agency within massive power relations] can be—however momentarily, however partially—held at bay."[68] Teenage enjoyment of ultragreasy bureks therefore, following Ortner, has less to do with the "agency

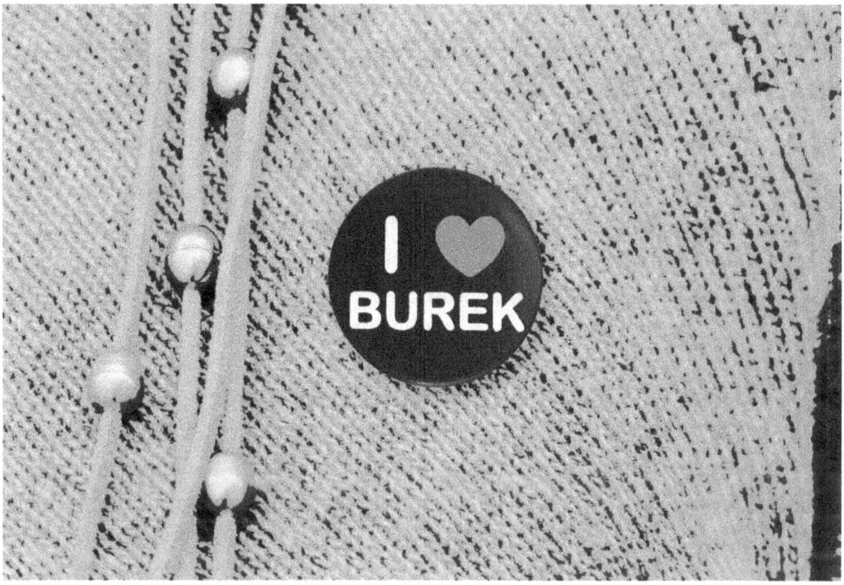

FIGURE 8.3 *A badge from Ljubljana streets. Photo © Jernej Mlekuž, Ljubljana 2016.*

of power" than with the "agency of projects": "[T]he first is organized around the axis of domination and resistance, and thus defined to a great extent by the terms of the dominant party, while the second is defined by the local logics of the good and the desirable and how to pursue them."[69] It has to do, to use Ortner's words again, with how students "seek to accomplish valued things within a framework of their own terms, their own categories of value."[70]

So that the paper will be more than just greasy

The taking of a subversive or at least somewhat ironic stance toward hegemonic healthy-lifestyle discourse in the context of the burek and its unhealthiness and greasiness can also be found outside of the secondary school milieu. Along with Foucault we could say that points of rebellion are present throughout networks of power. Lanko, the "ordinary guy but also a major burekologist," who is otherwise a lover and advocate of greasy bureks, when rating a squash burek from one of the Ljubljana bakeries, makes the following critical assessment: "The proximity of the hospital gives the burek shop an air of health or at least of healthcare ... which in my opinion is also the main reason that their bureks are not greasy."[71] But probably more than subversiveness, greasy bureks also offer adults the opportunity to escape the orderly world of duties, obligations, and rules. It opens up other "possibilities." In the Slovenian *Cosmopolitan*, in an insert called "Your Cosmo Guide to Contraception," we find the burek among the following "possibilities":

> Babies smell so nice: of apricots, organic diaper rash creams, and possibilities. But there is nothing wrong with wanting to inhale other pleasures at that moment: the smell of lime and tequila from happy margarita times, a dab of perfume before a date, or even a greasy burek and a coffee the following morning. This can also smell of possibilities.[72]

As Barthes says, "food serves as a sign not only for themes, but also for situations."[73] And the burek is also for adults a sign for situations that extend outside of duties, obligations, and rules. But let us return to young people and their burek eating. It is important to note that other meanings or aspects of rebellion are present in the appropriation of bureks by secondary schoolers and young people in general, which can in no way be sought in all situations, examples, and contexts. As I said above, high school burek eating is primarily about rebellion with and for the burek, and has to be understood as a sort of mélange of meanings, interests, and associations. As I said at the beginning of this chapter, their burek eating is probably to a great extent about one or another form of opposition to the dominant family structure of eating and the authority of adults (Figure 8.2). Even the act of eating an ultragreasy burek and making jokes at the expense of healthy-lifestyle discourse can be interpreted primarily as opposition to a discourse, which is imposed by the world of adults. The manner in which the burek is eaten—with the fingers, which are usually then cleaned by licking—can be interpreted as an act of rebellion against adult rules of decorum with regard to "proper" eating habits.[74] Certain statements by young burek eaters, for instance, counting the calories in an ultragreasy burek, can be explained not just as opposition to healthy-lifestyle discourse but also as opposition to ascetic imperatives by privileging pleasure and enjoyment. Food in this context seems not to be just a chemical mix of calories and dangers but is also an object of delight. In certain situations, contexts, and statements of young people in connection with bureks, it is also possible to detect opposition to "Americanization" or "McDonaldization," that is, opposition to standardized, rationalized, hegemonic American culture.[75] This shows up in several online debates, including one called "Burek vs. McDonald's."[76] Rejections of Yugophobia, Balkanophobia, and other nationalistic phenomena are also present in other online debates, comments, and statements, and in the title of a text called, "Burek bi, a džamije ne, a?" (You would like a burek, but not a mosque, eh?) on the website "Student Info," which developed into a heated debate.[77]

As stated in the introduction, in Slovenia today the burek is not just a signifier or metaphor of greasy and unhealthy food and not just a target of healthy-lifestyle discourse. The burek has acquired the status of some sort of strong, highly magnetized signifier, a metasymbol,[78] which is capable of attracting very different meanings and uses—most often, but in no way exclusively, nationalistic.[79] The omnipresence and multiplicity of meanings of the burek in Slovenian society and culture are illustrated by an enormous number of various phrasemes in Slovene relating to the burek. For instance, the phraseme "You're a burek," which is frequently heard primarily in slang, usually means an incompetent or an idiot. In this insulting use, the word "burek" can also imply a stupid and incompetent "southerner," a person from the Balkans, an immigrant. In contrast, among the teenage peer groups, this phraseme is often, but not always, used to express the exact opposite—a term of endearment. Social and cultural phenomena are quite a bit more complicated than our narrations about them, and quite a bit more confusing than our theories. As a result, the networks of various power and discourses are much more complex than researchers are able to present.

These symbolic meanings of the burek among secondary schoolers and young people in general also manifest in a wealth of (sub)cultural production: in very different textual forms, in various contexts in slang, in widely varying forms on websites, in jokes, gags, and stories. What do the scribbles below mean (Figure 8.4)?

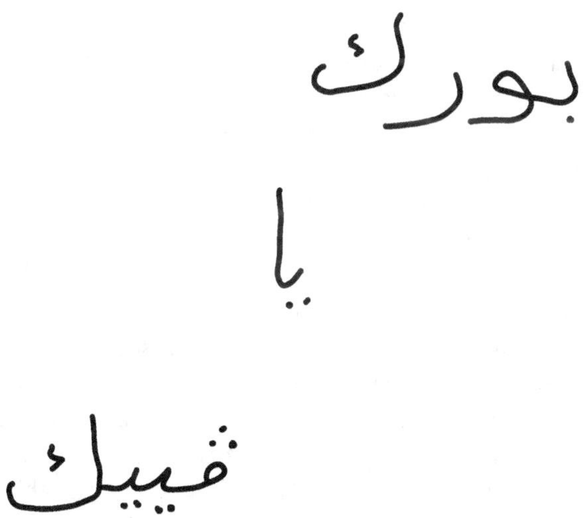

FIGURE 8.4 *"The Burek Is Great" in Arabic. Courtesy A. J.*

This is an Arabic inscription of "The burek is great," a paraphrase of "God/Allah is great," which we find on the home page of the website of Škofijska Gymnasium student A. J. He even named his server burek, so his e-mail address is mesni@burek.uni.cc (that is, "meat@burek.uni.cc").[80] He states, "Some [people who visited his website and enjoyed it] asked me for an e-mail address on my server, and of course they got them. Having a burek e-mail address is a real status symbol." In response to the question "Why burek?", he replies enigmatically, "maybe because I like to eat bureks:)."[81]

Conclusion or a few more greasy stains

In modern Slovenian society and culture, the burek is a signifier, which is frequently employed whenever people write, talk, or think about greasiness or fat, and particularly about greasy and unhealthy food. Healthy-lifestyle discourse, which is the primary culprit in the propagation, the emphasizing, and the ridiculing of the burek's greasiness, thus deals with and constructs the burek in a scientific, professional, and institutional, but even more in an imaginative, fictive, and notional sense. This, of course, does not mean that healthy-lifestyle discourse strictly determines what is possible to say about and do with the burek. But it does mean that a specific network of meanings, interests, connections, associations, truths, and self-evidence is often employed whenever bureks are spoken, written, and thought about, and when all manner of things are done with them.

The secondary school appropriation of the "ultragreasy" burek is also caught in this network of healthy-lifestyle discourse, and can be interpreted simply as rebellion against and a mocking of healthy-lifestyle discourse. But this eating of "ultragreasy" bureks, often seasoned with jokes at the expense of hegemonic healthy-lifestyle discourse, is above all and primarily a material practice, historically and geographically determined, and is thus embedded in the rhythm of everyday life and individual and social reproduction. A greasy burek eaten by a hungry secondary school student after a difficult class is (at least for the hungry secondary school student) not the same thing as the equation for the burek in which the greasiness is squared in the numerator. Secondary schoolers who eat ultragreasy bureks do not do so primarily and usually also not consciously in order to rebel against healthy-lifestyle discourse. They do so because bureks are cheap, nearly universally available, filling, eaten with the hands, and tasty. And they are probably even tastier because for the loudmouthed, irritating healthy-lifestyle discourse, the burek is a greasy lowlife. But in all of this it seems that more than opposition to and rebellion against healthy-lifestyle discourse is going on. It is about how students find and create spaces of autonomy and self-expression, or, in Ortner's words, how they "seek to nourish and protect by creating sites, literally or metaphorically, 'on the margins of power'."[82] Thus, still following Ortner, it is more about the "agency of projects" than the "agency of power."[83]

The greasy burek's greatest strength probably lies in the simple, banal material fact that it is filling, and that like it or not it leaves grease stains. In the case of secondary schoolers' eating of ultragreasy bureks, we have to turn Claude Lévi-Strauss's well-worn dictum on its head[84]: before the burek became good to think with, it had to be good to eat.

Notes

1 A modified version of this text was previously published in Croatian (Jernej Mlekuž, "Burek je mastan, ultramastan, velik: Uživanje bureka u nekim generacijskim skupinama u Sloveniji," *Etnološka Tribina* 36 (2013): 81–89), and some parts have been published in a book on the meanings of the burek; see Jernej Mlekuž, *Burek: A Culinary Metaphor* (Budapest: CEU Press, 2015).

2 The Carniolan burek was released onto the market in 2013 by the industrial food processing company and probably Slovenia's largest bakery, Žito, which states the following about its new product on its website: "Slovenia's favorite fast food with a traditional Slovenian taste is finally here!"; Žito, "kranjski burek," accessed May 13, 2016, http://kruh.zito.si/2013/05/kranjski/. The Slovenian colonization of the (Carniolan) burek is further decorated with the Slovenian flag, which is stuck into this "Carniolan" product. This move by Slovenia's largest baker was responded to by its largest competitor, Pekarna Pečjak, which in that same year spat the "gibanica burek" onto the market—a hybrid of a burek and one of the most representative Slovenian desserts.

3 But this mass presence and complex incorporation of the burek, cf. Dick Hebdige, *Subculture: The Meaning of Style* (London, New York: Methuen, 1979), still does not mean that all doors are open to the burek, much less wide open. But this is a story with another title.

4 Fionn Davenport, *Best of Ljubljana: The Ultimate Pocket Guide & Map* (London: Lonely Planet Publications, 2006).

5 Marshall Sahlins, *Waiting for Foucault, Still* (Chicago: Prickly Paradigm Press, 2002), 20.

6 Per Hergren, *Path of Resistance: The Practice of Civil Disobedience* (Philadelphia: New Society Publishers, 1993).

7 Douglas Kellner, *Media Culture: Cultural Studies, Identity and Politics between the Modern and the Postmodern* (London, New York: Routledge, 1995).

8 Lila Abu-Lughod, "The Romance of Resistance: Tracing Transformations of Power through Bedouin Women," *American Ethnologist* 17, no. 1 (1990): 41–5.

9 Anthony Giddens, *The Consequences of Modernity* (Cambridge: Polity Press, 1992); Ulrich Beck, *Risk Society: Towards a New Modernity* (London: SAGE, 1992).

10 This focus on personal survival strategies has its roots in the failing of the socialist state at the end of the 1980s, the lack of funds for social security and healthcare, and the associated urging by medical professionals and the state toward individual responsibility for health. See Kevin White, *An Introduction to the Sociology of Health and Illness* (London: SAGE, 2002), 53–77.

11 Giddens, *Consequences*, 102.

12 White, *Sociology of Health*, 43. According to Mennel, rather than explicitly medical reasons, the progressive move toward the "civilizing" of appetite (with emphasis on refinement and self-control as a sign of courtly manners) began to change dietary habits in Europe in the sixteenth and the seventeenth century. See Stephen Mennell, *All Manners of Food: Eating and Taste in England and France from the Middle Ages to the Present* (Oxford: Basil Blackwell, 1987).

13 Richard Gwyn, *Communicating Health and Illness* (London: SAGE, 2002); Clive Seale, *Media and Health* (London: SAGE, 2002).

14 White, *Sociology of Health*, 51.

15 See the chapters by Nina Mackert and Jürgen Martschukat for food practices of self-control.

16 Montanari writes about the importance and desirability of fats in the history of European nutrition. The last chapter begins with the thoughts of a French farmer from an eighteenth-century text: "If I were king, I would drink nothing besides grease." According to Montanari, this is also the source of the aesthetic ideal that fat is beautiful, a sign of wealth and nutritional well-being. The ideals of thinness appeared as a new aesthetic and cultural model only in the eighteenth century, among social groups (mostly urban) that opposed the "old regime" in support of new ideological and political points of view. Massimo Montanari, *The Culture of Food* (Oxford: Blackwell Publishers, 1996).

17 Deborah Lupton, *Food, the Body and the Self* (London: SAGE, 1996), 82; Lauren Williams and John Germov, "The Thin Ideal: Women, Food, and Dieting," in *A Sociology of Food and Nutrition: The Social Appetite*, ed. L. Williams and J. Germov (South Melbourne: Oxford University Press, 1999), 205–27 and 209; Montanari, *Culture of Food.*

18 See Lupton, *Food*, 80–2. Blanka Tivadar, who conducted an analysis of changes in discourses about healthy food over the period from 1949 to 1990 in Slovenia's leading women's magazine, *Naša Žena* [Our woman], showed that texts were appearing as early as the end of the sixties that mentioned the connection between excessive consumption of fats and sugar and cardiovascular diseases, diabetes, and premature mortality. *Naša žena* was also already writing at that time about the benefits of unsaturated fatty acids; Blanka Tivadar, "*Naša žena* med željo po limonini lupici in strahom pred njo: Zdrava prehrana v socializmu," *Družboslovne razprave* 61 (2009): 7–23. There are several, often interrelated reasons for the dramatic change from valorizing to demonizing fats. In addition to new nutritional and medical attitudes, and structural aspects such as food supply or price, it is also necessary to mention the new, changed valuation of fatness, which not only posited the new aesthetic ideal but also closely associated fatness with unhealthiness. Lupton, *Food*, thus speaks of the "food/health/beauty triplex." The modern antifat stance, which, as we have said, also hides to a great extent behind the antigreasy food stance, was accepted or foisted upon us in the 1970s by the medical establishment, state health-care and other authorities, and by the fashion industry. See Williams and Germov, "The Thin Ideal," 209. A similar fate was also experienced by numerous other nutritional elements and foods (sugar, white bread, and white food in general, which was still very highly valued in the 1960s). Of course, when making such generalizations, we cannot forget about social differences and influences. As Pierre Bourdieu observed, the bourgeoisie manifests "class racism which associates the populace with everything heavy, thick and fat"! Pierre Bourdieu, *Distinction: A Social Critique of the Judgement of Taste* (Cambridge, MA: Harvard University Press, 1984), 178.

19 Mlekuž, *Burek.*

20 The emphases in the quotations are my own unless otherwise indicated.

21 G. Vulić, "Mesni burek v prehrani, analiza kvalitete in predlog za izboljšanje" (BA diss., Biotechnical Faculty, Oddelek za živilstvo, University of Ljubljana, 1991), iii.

22 This exchange between scientific/professional and lay/imaginative meanings of the burek seems to be a rich, if not unavoidable one, but it is not a priori provable. In fact it is not, at least in my opinion, a democratic exchange. It is a relatively one-way move from "science" to the imaginative and fictive. However, it seems to me that it is important to reject any notion that it is possible to mechanically transfer the great facts and truths disseminated by medical and dietary "science" into the complex field of culture. "Scientific" interest turned the burek into unhealthy food, and culture then turned the burek into a complex and diverse object.

23 Franc Marušič, "Burek blog," accessed October 18, 2006, http://www.delo.si/blog/ivanmars/index.php?BLOG_PATH=220&BLOG_ARCHIVE.

24 A. Ž., e-mail to the author, March 31, 2005.

25 Mika, "(I Don't Know What's Going) On," *Blogspot.com*, October 13, 2013, accessed May 13, 2016, http://mikaswildmoodswing.blogspot.com/2013/10/nr21.html.

26 Afrodita, "SMS Diete: Ločevalna dieta," *Smsdieta.si*, February 26, 2007, accessed August 10, 2014, http://forum.smsdieta.si/discussion/53/4/locevalna-dieta/.

27 Marin Medak, "Kako mladino motivirati za aktiven življenjski slog?," *Marinmedak.com*, February 6, 2011, accessed August 10, 2014, http://www.marinmedak.com/hrvaska-rekord/kako-mladino-motivirati-za-aktiven-zivljenjski-slog.

28 M.B., "Revirji ujemi-spusti za lov krapa preteklost?," September 25, 2008, accessed August 10, 2014, http://ribici-slovenije.si/forum/viewtopic.php?f=11&t=5967&start=20.

29 Slepiurar, " 'Ješ burek??'," 2008, accessed May 13, 2016, http://www.genspot.com/blog-6040/jes-burek.aspx. The emphasis is added.

30 D. Zajec, "Krotilci tigrov v šolskih klopeh," *Delo*, September 4, 2000, 3.

31 "Katarina Čas. Ljubiteljica bureka in vampov," *Nova*, March 19, 2007, 49.

32 Jakob Klemenčič and Marcel Ruijters, back cover, in *Stripburek: Comics from Behind the Rusty Iron Curtain*, ed. Katarina Mirović et al. (Ljubljana: Forum Ljubljana, 2007), Stripburger.

33 D. Mal, "Obleka naredi vojaka," *Vecˇ*, February 6, 2004, 24. The emphasis is added.

34 Roland Barthes, "Toward a Psychosociology of Contemporary Food Consumption," in *Food and Culture*, ed. C. Counihan and P. Van Esterik (London, New York: Routledge, 1997), 20–35 and 25.

35 See Mlekuž, *Burek*.

36 Staša Grom, "Low fat sirov burek," April 17, 2006, accessed May 13, 2016, http://maxximum-portal.com/Recepti/Razno/17/32/265/17/Low_Fat_sirov_burek/.

37 The "political economy of truth" in modern societies is characterized, according to Foucault, by the following attributes: (1) truth depends on scientific discourse and the institutions that produce it; (2) it is subject to continuous political and economic stimulation; (3) it is defined extremely broadly and in consumerist terms (through educational and informational structures); (4) it is produced under the supervision of large political and economic structures (universities, the military, the media); (5) it is a subject of political debate and social confrontation (so-called ideological warfare). Cf. Michel Foucault, *Power/Knowledge: Selected Interviews and Other Writings, 1972–1977*, ed. Colin Gordon (New York: Pantheon Books, 1980), 131.

38 Foucault, *Power/Knowledge*, 131.

39 See the chapter by Nina Macket on the struggles for healthier selves.

40 Slepiurar, " 'Ješ burek??' "

41 Z. Kužet, " 'Moški vikend' v Ljubljani" ['Men's weekend' in Ljubljana,] *Večer*, October 5, 2005, 35.

42 Marušič, "Burek blog."

43 See Lupton, *Food*, 55–9. These include affinities to fast food, vegetarianism, and eating disorders. According to Deborah Lupton, growing girls and young women use food to express disagreement or rebellion, since they have fewer social resources at their disposal than men do.

44 See the chapter in this volume by Eva Barlösius for more on children, youth, and food.

45 Claude Fischler, "Learned versus 'Spontaneous' Dietetics: French Mothers' Views of What Children Should Eat," *Social Science Information* 25, no. 1 (1986): 945–65 and 950.

46 Cf. Nickie Charles and Marion Kerr, *Women, Food and Families* (Manchester, UK: Manchester University Press, 1988), 104–5.

47 Allison James, "Confections, Concoctions and Conceptions," in *Consumption: Objects, Subjects and Mediations in Consumption*, ed. D. Miller (London: Routledge 1982), 70–85 and 83.

48 Michel Foucault, "The Order of Discourse," in *Untying the Text: A Post-Structuralist Reader*, ed. R. Young (Boston: Routledge & Kegan Paul, 1981), 51–76 and 52–3.

49 Meta Medved et al., "Prehrambene navade ljubljanskih osmošolcev," *Zdravstveno varstvo* 37 (1998): 211–17 and 211.

50 A. J., e-mail to the author, March 21, 2005.

51 J. V., pers. comm., July 7, 2006

52 Ibid.

53 The study by Chapman and Maclean (cited in Lupton, *Food*, 58) on the eating habits of Canadian teenagers is interesting in this context. They associate eating unhealthy food with both positive (comfort, fun, socializing with friends, absence of parental authority) and negative elements (fatness, guilt, gluttony). Healthy food, in contrast, is associated with home, control of the body and body weight, care for one's appearance, and parental supervision. Despite their dietary awareness, they conceptualize unhealthy food as the norm, and healthy food as an oddity. The authors conclude that the association between independence, adolescent identity, and unhealthy food is stronger than the fear of being fat, which is also the case with burek-eating Slovenian secondary schoolers. Similarly, James, "Confections," in her study of children's sweets concludes that sweets are treated by children as a object of resistance to adult norms.

54 Cf. Stuart Hall, *Representation: Cultural Representations and Signifying Practices* (London: SAGE, 2002), 269–75.

55 Michel Foucault, "The Subject and Power," in *Michel Foucault: Beyond Structuralism and Hermeneutics*, ed. Hubert L. Dreyfus and P. Rabinow (New York: Harvester Wheatsheaf, 1983), 208–26 and 221.

56 Edward W. Said, *Orientalism* (London: Penguin, 2003).

57 Foucault, "The Subject and Power," 225.

58 Hebdige, *Subculture*.

59 We can hypothesize that bureks are filling precisely because they are greasy. At least that is how they are understood by burek eaters, including the burek assessor Lanko Marušič: "By late-night nutrition I have in mind suitably greasy, nearly transparent dough, which leaks so much oil into the paper that if you hold it wrong it likes to run directly towards innocent, unassuming sleeves or other parts of shirts, pullovers, jackets etc.," http://www.delo.si/blog/ivanmars/index.php?BLOG_PATH=220&BLOG_ARCHIVE.

60 M. Č., e-mail to the author, July 17, 2006.

61 Marx uses this sentence to explain the relationship between exchange value and abstract human labor. Thus he states, "whenever, by an exchange, we equate as values our different products, by that very act, we also equate, as human labor, the different kinds of labor expended upon them. We are not aware of this, nevertheless we do it." Karl Marx, *Capital: A Critique of Political Economy, vol. 1, The Process of Capitalist Production*, ed. Frederick Engels (Chicago: Charles H. Kerr and Co., 1909), 83.

62 See the chapters in this volume by Jürgen Martschukat for more on fit bodies and by Eva Barlösius for more on the stigmatization of fat bodies.

63 Hebdige, *Subculture*, 100ff.

64 In British subcultural styles, at least in Hebdige's time, this recontextualization of commodities and objects was most pronounced and noticeable in the clothing style of the punks. Objects from more banal contexts—toilet pull chains, pins, plastic bags, tampons, razor blades—became a part of their style; Hebdige, *Subculture*, 107 and passim.

65 Susan Seymour, "Resistance," *Anthropological Theory* 6, no. 3 (2006): 303–21 and 305. One undoubtedly important question in the understanding and conceptualization of rebellion is whether it has to be planned and intentional for us to be able to speak of rebellion at all. There are, of course, various points of view on how we can look at rebellion: Sherry B. Ortner, *Anthropology and Social Theory: Culture, Power, and the Acting Subject* (Durham, NC: Duke University Press, 2006); Jocelyn A. Hollander and Rachel L. Einwohner, "Conceptualizing Resistance," *Sociological Forum* 19, no. 4 (2004): 533–54, 537–8, and 544. However, despite the various definitions, there is a certain consensus that rebellion is always based on (a) action or active behavior (which can be verbal, cognitive, or physical) and (b) resistance, opposition, and defiant elements.

66 Eetaq, "Maturanc, EETAQ ali BEDA?," accessed May 13, 2016, http://www.eetaq.si/maturantski-zakljucni-ples-bonton-in-kaj-se-spodobi.

67 Ortner, *Anthropology*, 142

68 Ibid., 143.

69 Ibid., 145.

70 Ibid.

71 Marušič, "Burek blog."

72 P. Arula, "Tvoj cosmo vodnik po kontracepciji," *Cosmopolitan Slovenija*, March 3, 2015, 15.

73 Barthes, "Toward a Psychosociology," 25.

74 Cf. James, "Confections."

75 George Ritzer, *The McDonaldization of Society: An Investigation into the Changing Character of Contemporary Social Life* (Thousand Oaks, CA: Pine Forge Press, 1996).

76 Zygo, "Burek VS McDonald's."

77 S. Prajnić, "Burek bi, a đamije ne, a??," accessed July 13, 2006, http://www.student-info.net/portal/portal.php?stran=prva&vs=novice&id=173.

78 See Daniel Miller, "Coca-Cola: A Black Sweet Drink from Trinidad," in *Material Cultures: Why Some Things Matter*, ed. D. Miller (London: UCL Press, 1998), 169–87.

79 See Mlekuž, *Burek*.

80 A. J., 2005, "Burek je velik," accessed August 16, 2006, http://burek.uni.cc/.

81 A. J., e-mail messages to the author, March 21 and 22, 2005.

82 Ortner, *Anthropology*, 144.

83 Ortner, *Anthropology*.

84 Claude Lévi-Strauss, *Totemism* (London: Merlin Press, 1962), 89.

List of Contributors

Eva Barlösius is Professor of Macrosociology at the Leibniz University of Hannover and Head of the Leibniz Center for Science and Society (LCSS). Her areas of expertise include the sociology of eating, inequality, science studies, and rural areas.

Rossella Ceccarini holds a PhD in global studies from Sophia University, Tokyo. She is the author of *Pizza and Pizza Chefs in Japan: A Case of Culinary Globalization* (Leiden: Brill, 2011). She is interested in interdisciplinary and ethnographic research, cultural and food studies, sociology of work and occupations.

Nina Mackert is Assistant Professor of North American History at the University of Erfurt, where she obtained her PhD in History in 2012. Her dissertation on the US-American delinquency scare after 1945 was published in 2014 with UVK. Currently, she is writing a book about the history of the calorie in the United States. Recent publications include articles on the history of food, fat, ability, and subjectivation in the decades around 1900. She is the coeditor of the food studies blog foodfatnessfitness.com, and of "Fat Agency," a special issue of the journal *Body Politics* 5 (2015). Her recent research has been supported by the Fritz-Thyssen-Foundation and the VolkswagenStiftung.

Jürgen Martschukat is Professor of North American History at the University of Erfurt. He is the principal investigator of a research project on "The Eating Self," sponsored by the Fritz-Thyssen-Foundation, and member of an interdisciplinary research group on the history of "Food and Health in Modern Societies." His latest book on *Die Ordnung des Sozialen* (Frankfurt/M.: Campus, 2013) won the Adams Award of the Organization of American Historians and an award from Geisteswissenschaften International. He is currently working on a history of fitness.

Jernej Mlekuž is a research fellow at the Slovenian Migration Institute at the Research Centre of the Slovenian Academy of Sciences and Arts. He is the author of *Burek: The Culinary Metaphor* (Budapest: Central European University Press, 2015). Currently he is working on a study of kranjska klobasa—a sausage that played a significant role in the formation of Slovene consciousness from the spring of the nation onward.

Christoph Ribbat is a Professor of American Studies at the University of Paderborn (Germany). He is the author of *Flickering Light: A History of Neon* (London: Reaktion Books, 2013) and of a cultural history of the restaurant, forthcoming with Pushkin Press.

Keiichi Sawaguchi is Professor in the Faculty of Psychology and Sociology at Taisho University, Tokyo. His research interests center on the sociology of the family, profession, and life course, particularly on the change of career structure in specific industries and social contexts. His current research investigates the history of the restaurant industry in Japan and the life histories of restaurant workers. His most recent article is entitled "Japanese Cooks in Italy: The Path-Dependent Development of a Culinary Field," in *The Globalization of Asian Cuisines* (New York: Palgrave Macmillan, 2015).

Leonard Schmieding is a historian and studies entanglements between America and Germany in popular, consumer, and everyday culture. His first book, *"Das ist unsere Party": HipHop in der DDR* (Stuttgart: Steiner, 2014) examined hip-hop culture in the German Democratic Republic. Currently, he is writing a book about San Francisco Germans and the cultural work of their immigrant food cultures at the Golden Gate during the late nineteenth and early twentieth centuries.

Bryant Simon is Professor of History at Temple University and the cofounder of the *What is Your Food Worth?* Project. He is the author of *Everything But the Coffee: Learning about America from Starbucks* (Berkeley: University of California Press, 2009). Currently he is writing a book about chicken tenders, deregulation, and the hidden and high costs of cheap food. His recent research has benefitted from the general support of the Alexander von Humboldt Foundation.

Index

Page numbers in italics refer to figures.

www.ingramcontent.com/pod-product-compliance
Lightning Source LLC
LaVergne TN
LVHW052322200926
848481LV00002B/639